Perimenopause and Menopause:

What you really want to know,
but no one tells you.

ECLIPSED
INK

For Jesse and Liv,
Thanks for being my biggest supporters and
accepting me for me - hot flashes, mood swings, and all.

Thank you to my girls, my "beta readers," my tribe,
for your time, knowledge, encouragement, and
years of friendship. I'm lucky to have you.

And thanks to my parents for their unwavering love.
Skip any section on sex or with the word "vagina."
I don't want the holidays to be awkward.

PERIMENOPAUSE

and Menopause

What you really want to know,
but no one tells you.

ANGIE SCHWENDEMAN

contents

70
WTF IS GOING ON
WITH MY FACE?

84
DID I JUST PEE
MYSELF?

97
DO I NEED WEIGHT
WATCHERS?

109
WHY DOES MY VAGINA
FEEL LIKE SANDPAPER?

118
FIND MY PHONE

132
HEAD, SHOULDERS,
KNEES AND TOES

140
HELLO 2AM

157
IS MY PHONE FONT
ABNORMALLY LARGE?

163
WHY DO I CRY
AT EVERYTHING?

177
HORMONE
REPLACEMENT?

193
THAT CAN'T
BE GOOD

198
WHERE ARE
MY TWEEZERS?

Alright ladies (and gentlemen)... Here I am, at the ripe age of 47, and my body is revolting against me. Why, you ask?

PERIMENOPAUSE

First, I suppose I need to give you my disclaimer. I am not a nurse, a doctor, a paramedic, or anything in the medical field. I am a woman, a mom, a wife, a photographer, and occasionally a writer. These experiences are my own. I decided to write this because in the beginning of this journey, I was clueless! Not to mention, people are sometimes hush-hush about the subject. Why is that?

Here's the thing - I am going to give you the ugly truth because you deserve it. Perimenopause is so much more than hot flashes!

P.S. This era of my life has turned me into a woman who curses. Consider yourself warned.

Medical Disclaimer: This book cannot and does not contain medical advice. The medical information is provided for general informational and educational purposes only and is not a substitute for professional medical advice.

01

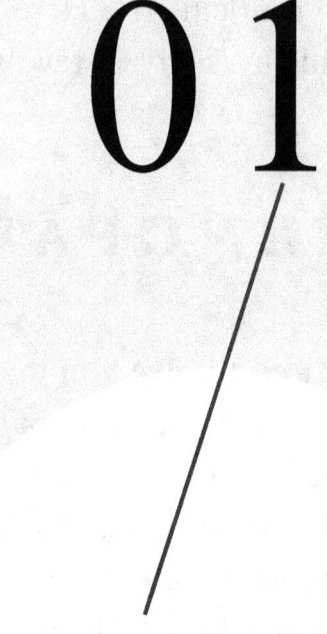

CHAPTER

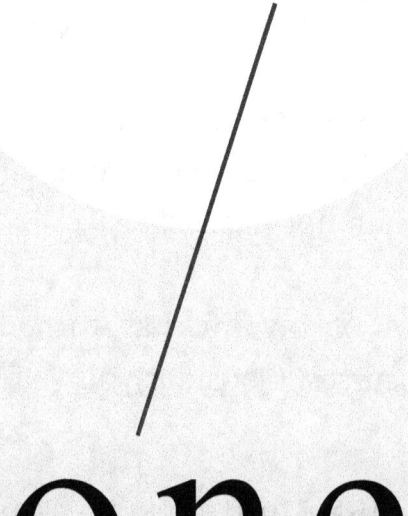

one

Chapter One
You're too young for this!

There I was in 2018 - 41 years old - headed to the gyno for my annual. This year was different because my periods were not normal. Far from it! When I say abnormal, I mean that some months I was having them every 2 weeks.

Side note - Welcome to my first side note! One of the lovely side effects of Perimenopause is brain fog. For me, it is less brain fog, and more brain-scatter. Now, before you jump to conclusions and tell me I am lucky to be going through "the change" so early, just hold on right there. While friends were having 3 and 4-day periods, mine lasted 8 days. That's not lucky - that is torture!

My ob-gyn history is pretty simple. I started my period at 14, and I've always had long periods. I wasn't on birth control or any hormone supplements. My cycles were always regular. In my early 20s, I was diagnosed with HPV, which led to one or two irregular Pap smears. Other than that, everything was normal - well, normal for me. At 32, I had my first and only child (her name's Liv, by the way). Fast forward to 41, and I'd had relatively no problems "down there."

Side note - For the gentlemen readers, a Pap smear is a procedure that collects and tests cervical cells for abnormality.

I clearly remember hearing the statement,
"You're too young for this!"
My gynecologist was a middle-aged woman,
perhaps ten years older than me. Then she started
rapid-firing all of the questions.

Side note - Didn't I already answer most of these questions
in the overly long, check-in paperwork you had me fill out?

"How long have your periods been like this?"
(answer - on and off for 6 months)
"When did your mother go through Menopause?"
(answer - she was 48)
"Are your cycles still normal, other than the time
between them?"
(answer - yes)
"Any other symptoms?"
(answer - not that I know of?)
Then she said it again,
"You're too young for this!"
"I'm too young for what?" I knew the answer, but I
NEEDED to hear it.

"PERIMENOPAUSE"

There it was. She said it. *Fuck.*
"Okay, what's next?" I asked nervously.

Her answer wasn't really an answer. I needed to get some bloodwork done and make sure my thyroid and other levels were normal. *They were.* I had an ultrasound on my ovaries and uterus, and other stuff down there, to make sure they were functioning properly. *They were.* After that, it was a wait-and-see game, unless I wanted to get on birth control *I didn't.*

The next year continued with extremely long and irregular periods. My poor husband thought I was a constant trickle of blood. He wasn't wrong about the constant - he was very wrong about the trickle. It was more like a gush, a crimson tidal wave.

The first day of my now 8-day cycle was nothing much. The period was there, but hardly noticeable. Day two opened the floodgates and they stayed open for three more days. During that time, it was difficult to sleep because I would go through 2 tampons every 4-5 hours. Here's the nasty truth of it all...Yes, I put two super plus tampons in to stop the flooding. One lasted an hour or two tops! Let's be brutally honest - who has time to go to the bathroom every two hours? Not me.

It wasn't just heavy. It was clotty. I didn't have any cramping, just a few backaches.

Now, when you have big clots, you start to panic. Ready for some nasty stuff? These clots were the size of a silver dollar. Am I aging myself by that reference? I'm pretty confident millennials have no idea what a silver dollar even is!

Think this size... and larger. Here's another little fact that no one told me... when you're on your period, the tampon won't absorb those lots - they just hang out on the outside and try to push your tampon out. Fantastic, isn't it?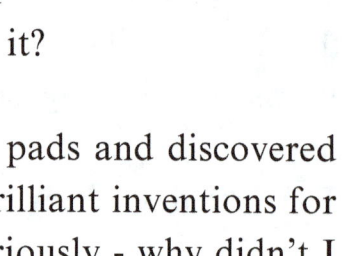

I started stockpiling jumbo pads and discovered probably one of the most brilliant inventions for women - period undies. Seriously - why didn't I think of that?!

Okay, okay, I digress. Let's get back to "You are too young for this" discussion. After talking about the next steps, I was more confused than ever. I also had the sneaking suspicion that my doctor did not think this was Perimenopause. Spoiler alert – it was. It was at that point, walking out of the doctor's office, that my journey truly began.

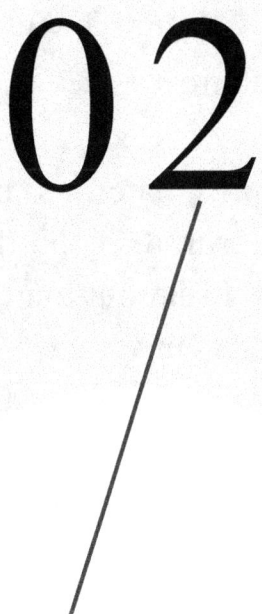

CHAPTER

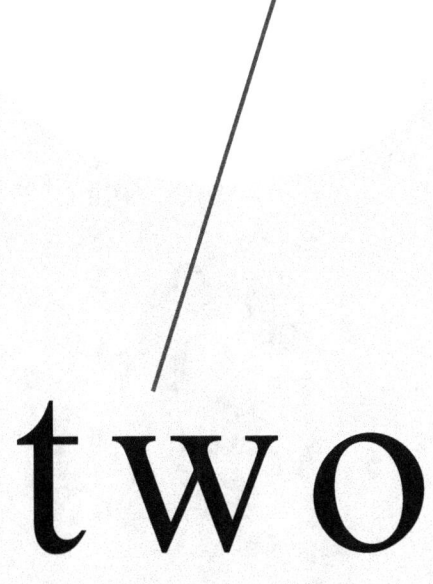

Chapter Two
Does anyone know a good Cardiologist?

About two months later, after the shocking gynecological visit, shit really hit the fan.

"What was that?!" I said out loud, to absolutely no one. I was standing in my kitchen, minding my own business, when my chest did a little... hiccup, or something.

"That was weird," I thought to myself.

Side note – I've always felt like I was in tune with my body. I could feel my period coming from a mile away. When I was sick, I knew whether I needed to go to the doctor and get antibiotics, or if it was a viral infection. And when I took a tumble, I knew it wasn't just a fall - I had actually snapped a couple of ligaments.

But this... This was different.
There it was again!
What the hell is going on in my chest??

Curiosity quickly turned into worry. Worry turned into panic. I started hearing my heartbeat. It seemed like it was beating out of my chest. Then the Googling began.

Typing...

```
What does a heart attack feel like?
Symptoms of a panic attack?
```
I've never had one and this was NOT one.
```
Why does my heart feel like it's
hiccupping in my chest?
```
Frantically typing...
```
What does it feel like when your
heart skips a beat?
```
Deep breaths, in and out. An hour had passed since the first episode. By then, I'd had two more, making it a total of three.

Call the husband.

"Hey... I'm not sure if everything is all right. Something's going on with my heart, or my chest, or something."

I tried to calmly explain it to him. Even over the phone, he heard through my attempt at calm. He could definitely tell that I was in freak-out mode.

"Go to Urgent Care. Now."

He was right. I should go. I gathered my stuff, collected my emotions, and hopped in the car.

The closest Urgent Care was only five minutes from my house. I could feel my heart racing, probably due to anxiety. Since the first episode of whatever the chest-hiccup was, I'd felt it several more times. After my earlier frantic Googling, I knew it sounded like I was having arrhythmias.

Side note – a heart arrhythmia is an irregular heartbeat. An arrhythmia occurs when the electrical signals that tell your heart to beat do not work properly. The heart may beat too fast or too slow. The pattern of the heartbeat may be inconsistent. An arrhythmia may feel like a fluttering, pounding, or racing heartbeat. Some arrhythmias are harmless. Others may cause life-threatening symptoms.

I consider myself a decent speller, but the word arrhythmia is the exception. Spellcheck for the win.

I'm not going to lie... I was scared shitless. I walked into the Urgent Care, taking note that the waiting room was practically full. I quickly walked to the sign-in area. Like normal, they asked for my insurance card, and if I'd been here before.

Side note - I had. Long story. Broken thumb. Not at all Perimenopause related.

Then the receptionist, who must've sensed my stress and worry, asked why I was there today?

"I think I'm having irregular heartbeats."

She immediately looked up and said,

"Okay, someone will be with you shortly."

I went to sit down in one of the few vacant chairs. As soon as my butt hit the plastic cushion, someone came out and called my name.

Side note – At an Urgent Care (and probably a hospital), if you tell them you have, or think you're having irregularities in your heart, they will immediately take you back to a room.

So, in I went. The nurse quickly took my vitals. I didn't step on the scale. *Thank goodness for small mercies.* Heart rate was slightly elevated at 95 bpm. My blood pressure was normal at 110/70.

A minute later, another nurse came in with a portable device. I quickly learned that the device was an EKG machine.

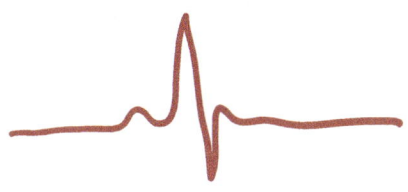

Side note – an electrocardiogram – an ECG or EKG measures the electrical activity of a heartbeat. With each heartbeat, an electrical impulse (or wave) travels through the heart. This electrical wave causes the muscles to squeeze and pump blood from the heart. A normal heartbeat on EKG will show the rate and rhythm of the contractions in the upper and lower chambers. The right and left atria (or upper chambers) make up the first wave, called the P wave – followed by a flat line when the electrical impulses go to the bottom chambers (or ventricles). The right and left bottom chambers make up the next wave, called a QRS complex. The final wave, or T wave represents electrical recovery or return to a resting state for the ventricles.

https://cpr.heart.org/en/health-topics/heart-attack/diagnosing-a-heart-attack/electrocardiogram-ecg-or-ekg

That's a lot of medical jargon, I know! In layman's terms, blood flows in and out of the four chambers, and the different waves show it's doing so at a normal (or abnormal) rate and rhythm.

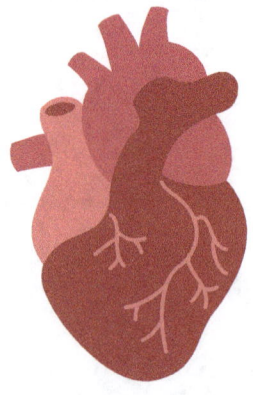

The nurse hooked me up to the portable EKG by attaching 5 sticky electrode patches to my chest. The machine did what is called a rapid EKG. The EKG prints out like a long receipt of your heart waves.

The doctor came in within five minutes of those tests. During that time, a nurse took a couple of vials of my blood to test for different cardiac enzymes.

The Doc was an older gentleman with salt-and-pepper hair and glasses. He shook my hand and introduced himself as Dr. So-and-so. He warmed up his hands and took my pulse.

"So, what's going on?"

I started from the beginning, doing my best to explain exactly what I was experiencing.

"Well, the good news is, your vitals are normal. Your heart rate is a little high, but that's to be expected with something like this. The bad news is that whatever is going on with your heart did not show up on the EKG. It's tough to catch arrhythmias because they are random, and we just took a three-minute snapshot of your heart. That snapshot looks normal."

I asked him, "Next steps?"

"There are certain things that trigger arrhythmias. Stress. Caffeine. Sometimes allergies. Having high blood sugar. Having sleep apnea. Smoking. And sometimes viral illnesses can disrupt your heart signals."

"So, I should stay away from those things?" I said sarcastically.

Side note - I tend to make jokes when I'm stressed.

He continued by telling me that I was immediately in need of a cardiologist.

"We can send an expedited referral over so they can see you sooner rather than later. In the meantime, try to relax. If you feel any sort of chest pain or pressure, go directly to the ER or call 911."

He shook my hand, wished me well, gave me a stack of papers, and told me to head up to check out. I was able to get into the cardiologist three days later.

I was content with this visit because I was convinced the doctor would call me crazy. He did ask if I had panic attacks (again, no!). He listened, took his time, and made me feel at ease.

I don't know about you, Reader, but there have been certain times in my life when I HATED going to the doctor. Here's my rank of doctor visits I would rather not do: 1) Gyno 2) Mammogram 3) Dermatologist 4) Cardiologist. As much as I know it's necessary, I still hate going to the doctor. Try to imagine my utter joy when I went to that heart appointment! I sincerely hope you are catching my deep sarcasm because going to the cardiologist that day was the last thing I wanted to do.

Side note - Do I have a fear of doctors? I don't think so. Did I fear that something was horribly wrong? 100%!

As I walked into my cardiologist's office, I couldn't help noticing that the waiting room was full of older men. I didn't realize it until I sat down, but something felt out of place. I think it was in my head, but I swear I could feel judgy glances.

Side note - I know I was being hypersensitive and over-paranoid, but I still felt out of place. I could feel my tension rise. Breathe in, counting to 4. Hold it for a four-count. Slowly breathe out, counting to 4. This is called Box Breathing. It calms my nerves.

Side note - Lots of side notes! Stress was definitely a trigger for my arrhythmias. When I would feel myself getting overly stressed, I would feel my heart palpitate. It was followed up by an episode.

In the hopes of witnessing the arrhythmias, I also bought myself a stethoscope from Amazon. I don't know if it was curiosity or obsession, but I was bound and determined to catch these arrhythmias in real life. And did I ever!

Here are my findings... My heart would beat fast (usually 4 beats, like 1234), then my heart would pause for one or two seconds, and then it would go back into regular rhythm. It's like my heart would skip a beat. When my heart would go back into sinus rhythm, I would feel a thump in my chest. Needless to say, it was such a strange feeling. I estimated that I would have one or two arrhythmias per hour.

The waiting room was typical. I think I waited about 45 minutes to see the doc. After what seemed like forever, a nurse took me back and put me in a room. From there, she put 12 electrodes on my chest and took a longer EKG. It might have lasted five minutes? Of course, I didn't feel a single arrhythmia during that time.

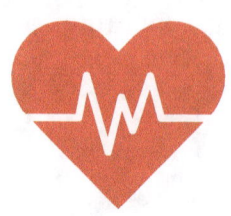

A young doctor (probably my age) came in and started asking me standard questions: What's going on? When did it begin? What are your symptoms? Has anything changed in your life?

"The only thing that has definitely changed is that I'm beginning to go through Perimenopause."

"That shouldn't be a factor," he quickly said.

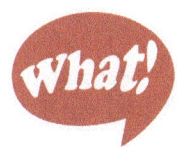

"Seriously?!" I asked with fervor. He then went on to tell me that fluctuations in hormones can cause palpitations but rarely arrhythmias.

Get a vagina and then answer that question. **But** of course, I didn't say that. I just sat there and listened.

Side note - To be fair, I feel like a female doctor would have been more understanding.

We chatted for a while and he explained my EKG, which at the time was normal. He did mention that the QT wave was slightly irregular. He then took a listen to my heart, from different placements on my chest, asking me to breathe normally and then breathe deep. Out of nowhere, it happened. *It* being an arrhythmia.

"That was it, wasn't it?" He asked me in such a casual tone.

"Yup!" I was actually excited that he caught the arrhythmia. I felt thankful and validated.

Side note - Up until that point, I knew for certain that something was physically going on with me. But was I going crazy?

"Okay - I caught the tail end of it. There are many different types of arrhythmias. Some are more serious, like A-fib, and some are minor and of little concern. What we need to find out is how often they are occurring."

"And... how do we do that?"

He continued, "I'd like you to wear a heart monitor for several weeks. It will record your heart and give us a clear idea of what is going on. I also want to run a few more blood tests."

"Anything else?" I asked.

He explained that I would get the monitor today and it starts recording today. In 14 days, I take it off and send it back to the manufacturer who will extract the information and send it to the cardiologist.

"Let's do it," I managed to say.

At the time, those two weeks went by SO slowly. Having a heart monitor on, although not invasive, was a pain in the ass. You could shower, but you had to tape it up and make sure it was covered completely so it did not get wet.

I was embarrassed to have sex. It may sound silly, but if the device was recording my heartbeats, it would register when my heart rate was... excited.

The last five days were the worst because the patch was itchy, and the adhesive was starting to peel off. But I made it through! I sent it back with expedited shipping. The doc explained there would be a little bit of a delay between when the manufacturer receives the machine, and when he gets the data. Because of that, I had to wait another two weeks for my follow-up appointment.

In the meantime, a funny thing happened... I started to get used to the arrhythmias. It's like they became a part of me. I would still feel them, but I wouldn't feel the amount of stress that I previously had felt. I was impatiently waiting for answers.

Side note - I hate the waiting game.

In those two weeks, I learned more about the heart, from my own research, than I ever did in any of my Anatomy and Physiology courses.

At the follow-up cardio appointment, I found out that I have a minor heart condition called SVT. Super Ventricular Tachycardia is a type of irregular heartbeat, also called an arrhythmia.

Side note - SVT is caused by faulty signaling in the heart. Oftentimes, an extra pathway causes this. The electrical signals in the heart control a heartbeat. In SVT, a change in the heart signaling causes the heartbeat to start too early in the atria. When that happens, the heartbeat speeds up, to catch up. That's what was happening to me.
I would, and still have a rapid heartbeat of five or six beats. After those fast beats, my Sinoatrial (SA) node, which is a part of the heart that acts like an internal pacemaker, would kick me into regular rhythm. The whole feeling is very bizarre, like an out-of-body experience. Perimenopause is like that isn't it? It's an out-of-body shitshow.

The doctor was unsure of what triggered these events. He did assure me that arrhythmias are not concerning when they are happening less than one percent of the heartbeats in a day.
Our hearts beat approximately 100,000 times a day. One Percent of that is 1000.

My doctor showed me the reports. There were a few days that I had more events than others. The most I had in one day was 96 times. My average per day was around 20 to 30.

He wasn't concerned and he said I shouldn't be concerned. For the two years following that appointment, I would see him every six months. After those two years, it turned into an annual visit.

Side note – As I journeyed through Perimenopause, my number of arrhythmias would fluctuate from week to week, and month to month. Some months, they were hardly noticeable at all. As I got inched closer to actual Menopause, the arrhythmias happened less and less.

I liked my cardiologist. He was kind and answered all of my questions. He was patient with me, and he tried to explain things while easing my fears. Even as I continue to see him, year after year, he still speaks as if hormones could not possibly be the cause of this. I just disagree.

I'm no doctor, but I do believe that my hormones, or lack thereof, had a hand in these arrhythmias. I'm sure of it. I'll stand by that belief because I was living proof.

I spoke to my gynecologist about it, and she laughed and said, "Cardiologists believe everything has to live and die with the heart. I would argue that hormones control so much more than we can scientifically prove."

When I asked her if she thought my arrhythmias might have been caused by my changing hormones?

She said, "Absolutely!"

Ladies! You are smart. Trust your instinct. Advocate for yourself. If you know something is wrong and a doctor dismisses you, find a doctor who will listen.

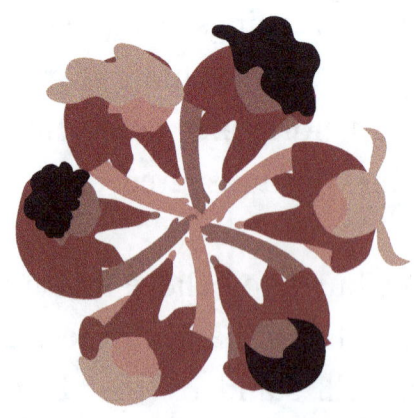

03

CHAPTER

three

Chapter Three
Let's call her Peri.

Let's not sugarcoat things... Peri's a bitch.

So, what's the difference between Peri and Meno? Growing up, and even until my late 30s - I had never heard of Peri! I find this odd because she certainly makes her presence known.

But why is that? I would like to consider myself a fairly intelligent person, but this baffles me! Are there things we just don't talk about? Is the subject too uncomfortable and women hide from it? Is Perimenopause taboo, or are there so many symptoms of Peri that it's hard to know where to begin?

Back to my first question... What is the difference between Perimenopause and Menopause? **Perimenopause is a transitional time that ends in Menopause.** Menopause means your periods have ended. When you have no menstrual cycle for a full 12 months, you have officially reached Menopause.

Seems simple enough?
Wrong! It's not simple at all.

This chapter is going to be more introductory. There are so many symptoms and so little time. After doing a ton of research, some of these Peri symptoms are downright bizarre!

Before sitting down to write this book, I read a lot about hormones and Perimenopause. I talked to friends, nurses, and doctors to get their input. Here's the funny thing... Everyone spoke differently, based on their experience and knowledge. There was one common thread, hormones wreak havoc on the body when they are not regulated, especially when they are in decline.

OK, so that adds up.

Peri is basically the gradual decline of estrogen and progesterone. It's the big drop in estrogen that really causes the most problems. Peri sticks around too. She can last up to 10 years.

These are the common symptoms, in a little game I just made up, called *This or That: Perimenopause Edition.*

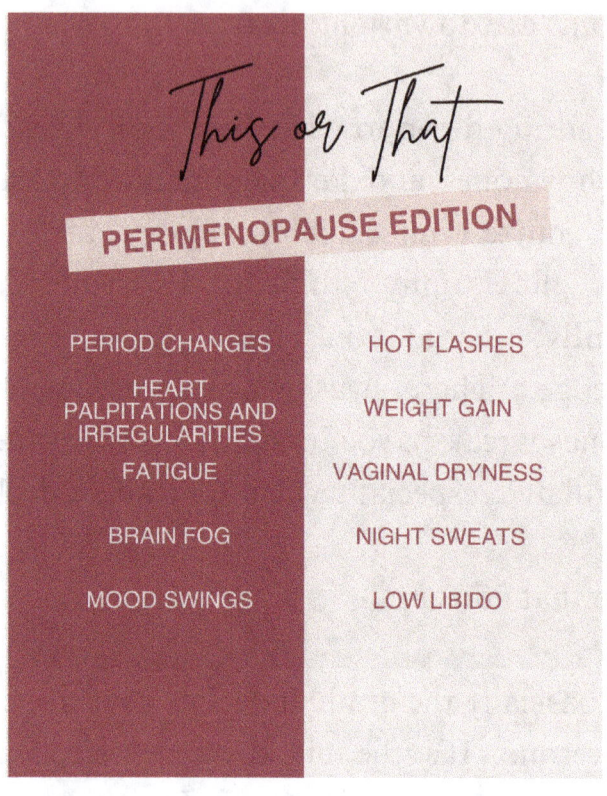

There are so many other random and wacky symptoms. We'll get to those in a minute!

I can tell you from personal experience, I experienced 9 out of 10 of these. Before you get scared, my symptoms were minor. I knew they were happening, but they didn't interrupt my life enough to make them major.

I still can't believe that in my circle - friends, parents, colleagues, social media, and even random internet reels - no one talks about this.

Before you get on my mom's case, stop right there. She didn't know, because she never experienced the majority of these symptoms.

Knowing when your mother and even grandmother were in Meno is pretty important. It's simply a good estimation of when you will go through it. My mom was 48 when she was completely done with her period. She was young, thank goodness for me. As I sit here and edit this, I am 47 years old, and I've been in active Meno for 1 month.

Want to know what the difference was between my mom and me? Birth control. Mom was on birth control until her periods began to stop. She didn't know it at the time, but that influx of hormones balanced the estrogen and progesterone scales. It was enough to keep her Peri symptoms minimal.

I stopped birth control in my mid to late 20s because I didn't like it. I also wanted to keep things as natural as possible. I genuinely wanted to know that my body/period was working without the added hormones.

I am also a bit of a stubborn, masochistic, dumbass.

Yes, I said that.

I knew I was struggling but kept doing it. I told myself... this is normal.

But what if it's not?

Side note - This doesn't need to turn into a self-psychoanalysis. I'm no Sigmund Freud.

So... the other symptoms - the ones that people really don't talk about... bloating, visceral fat, incontinence, joint pain, wrinkles, acne, facial (chin) hair, dry eyes, headaches, bleeding and gum sensitivity, digestive issues, etc.

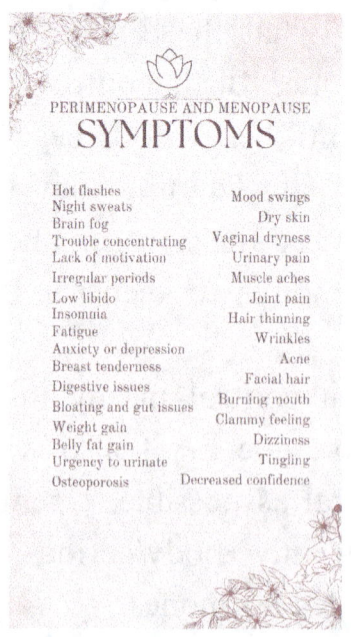

PERIMENOPAUSE AND MENOPAUSE
SYMPTOMS

Hot flashes
Night sweats
Brain fog
Trouble concentrating
Lack of motivation
Irregular periods
Low libido
Insomnia
Fatigue
Anxiety or depression
Breast tenderness
Digestive issues
Bloating and gut issues
Weight gain
Belly fat gain
Urgency to urinate
Osteoporosis

Mood swings
Dry skin
Vaginal dryness
Urinary pain
Muscle aches
Joint pain
Hair thinning
Wrinkles
Acne
Facial hair
Burning mouth
Clammy feeling
Dizziness
Tingling
Decreased confidence

Let's go deeper down this rabbit hole, shall we?
Looking at the longer list, those seem fairly
common. The next list, I have deemed to be the
WTF list...

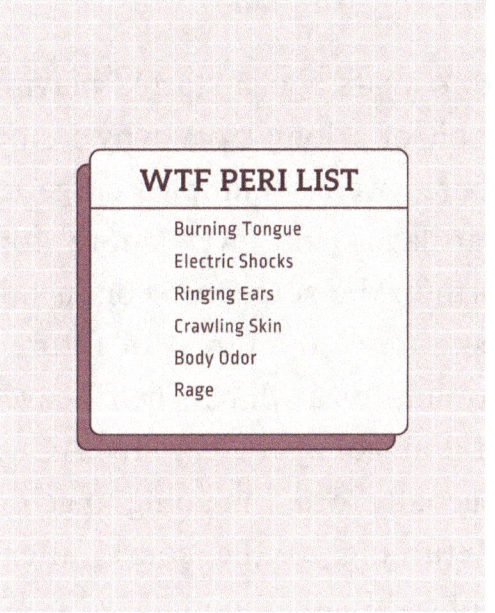

WTF PERI LIST

Burning Tongue
Electric Shocks
Ringing Ears
Crawling Skin
Body Odor
Rage

Burning tongue?!
Crawling skin?!
Electric shocks?!
No, thank you! I personally haven't experienced
these symptoms, but others aren't as lucky.

As far as ringing ears, body odor, and rage - I can
easily check the YES box for those.

Body odor...

Oh my, do I stink!

My husband can attest to this.

And here's a little TMI, I stink downstairs too.

Two years ago, I started playing tennis again. It's a bit of a long story why I stopped, let's just say there were multiple surgeries, multiple torn cartilage, and even more torn ligaments. My orthopedic surgeon recommended that I not play because of the threat of future injuries. I listened to him for a while. Then I caved and said fuck it. If I'm going to tear my ACL, which is already partially torn, I'm going to go down swinging.

Returning to the court, after decades away, I noticed I sweat more. My hubby also told me that I smell.

Insert RAGE Emoji 😡

He wasn't saying it to be mean. He's a very kind and pragmatic guy. He simply meant that I smell different.

"Do I smell?"

"Not necessarily. You just smell... ripe and sweaty, but not stinky." He responded, knowing that he was on thin ice.

So, that was an adjustment. I tried different deodorants, natural and unnatural, spray, gel, and even the white cakey stuff.

Google search – is antiperspirant bad for you?

Side note – it's 66 in my house, and I am currently having a hot flash. I was freezing a minute ago.

My Google search brought mixed reviews. I've also discovered people like to post very non-educated and non-scientific beliefs all over the Internet.

I won't rain on anyone's parade and tell them their opinion is wrong. It's not.

I will simply tell you my experience. I tried the natural, nontoxic deodorants - No aluminum, no parabens, and all of that stuff. They don't work for me. I wish they did.

After trying a handful or two of antiperspirants, I opted to stick with my original, Secret Outlast, Clear Gel. It works for now.

When I started playing more tennis, I quickly noticed that my boob sweat quadrupled. I deemed myself, the sweaty girl. My initial remedy was to put antiperspirant underneath my breasts.

CAUTION

This was wrong on so many levels. First and foremost, sweating is our body's natural way of regulating temperature. The first time I swiped antiperspirant under my tatas, something happened. In the middle of a match, I felt like I was going to internally combust. Was it the additional antiperspirant? Was it a hot flash? Was it a mixture of the two? I don't know, but I felt like I was going to pass out - and nearly did.

OK... So, I won't be doing that again.
Here's what works for me:
I can't stop the boob sweat, but I can wear a sports bra that goes a little bit lower on my chest.

I wear lots of Nike Dri-FIT tank tops. They seem to show the least amount of sweat and are quick to dry.

I have tons of sweat towels, and I use them. For the extremely hot days, I pack a cooling towel. Occasionally placing the cold towel on my neck works wonders, cooling me down immediately.

I'm sure you've seen the full-body deodorants, like Lume. I've never tried it, but a few friends swear by it. Lume comes in a spray, cream, solid, and body wipes.

I started wearing an additional, good-smelling deodorant, on top of the antiperspirant. It smells like Georgia peaches. I wear it under the boobs and between the legs.

Do keep in mind that antiperspirants and deodorants are very different.

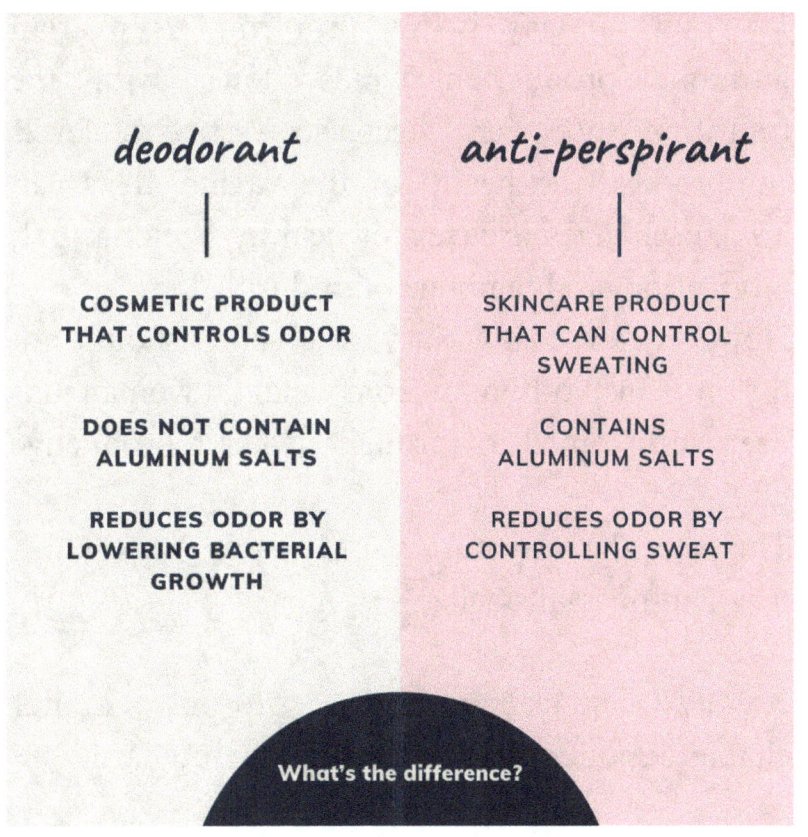

deodorant

COSMETIC PRODUCT
THAT CONTROLS ODOR

DOES NOT CONTAIN
ALUMINUM SALTS

REDUCES ODOR BY
LOWERING BACTERIAL
GROWTH

anti-perspirant

SKINCARE PRODUCT
THAT CAN CONTROL
SWEATING

CONTAINS
ALUMINUM SALTS

REDUCES ODOR BY
CONTROLLING SWEAT

What's the difference?

Want to know what else I do? I have a dress rehearsal. I hate being the sweaty girl, So, I do something at my house - workout, run for 60 seconds, just go outside on a summer's day, simply to test the functionality and sweatproof ability of a shirt. I even do this to test my pants. You sweat more down there too. It's awesome. By awesome, I mean awful. Did you think the term "swamp-ass" was just for men? It's not.

The stink can be from a couple of things.
1. Your vajayjay is the problem. As ovarian hormone production winds down with the transition into Peri, decreased estrogen levels compromise the health of the vagina. This can lead to changes in levels of healthy bacteria, pH, lubrication, and feminine odor during Peri.
However, the change in vaginal smell should not be foul, just different from what a woman has been accustomed to throughout her reproductive life.
This was the case for me. My lady parts had a new, but normal smell.

2. Mild Urine leakage - we'll get to this in a later chapter. Spoiler alert... Don't sneeze too hard.

The last reason is my most noticeable reason.

3. Hyperhidrosis - Hyperhidrosis is a medical condition that causes excessive amounts of sweating when the body does not need cooling.

Many women who suffer from hyperhidrosis, sweat excessively from only one or two areas of the body, which include the head, underarms, palms, groin, or feet. The rest of the body remains dry.

Yep, that's me.

It's really not the end of the world. Here's what I do about it. I shower, a lot. I do wear the natural peach deodorant down there - I swipe the groin and inner thigh before I play tennis or work out.

Side note - a deodorant helps odor but doesn't keep you from sweating. An antiperspirant controls the sweat. Sweating is normal and natural!

Do keep in mind - I only over-sweat while playing a sport. I think you all are picturing me, sitting at my computer, typing away, sweaty and stinky.

It's not that drastic.

The other random symptoms are rage and tinnitus (ringing ears).

Rage? Seriously? I really think this is an unfair symptom. What woman doesn't have rage? I think it's high time that we stop blaming women's anger on their hormones. Sometimes, we're just angry...

Angry at our husbands/partners for doing dumb things. (Honey, if you're reading this, I love you so very much, but you do some idiotic stuff that I don't understand).

You might be pissed because your child/children aren't listening.

You might be overly irritated in traffic because people are blowing their horns. Seriously, what's the point?

You might be furious because the neighbor's delinquent boys haphazardly hopped your fence and broke it for the second time in two months. "But they were just getting the basketball in your yard," says their mother. Insert more rage.

You might be seeing red because your mixed doubles tennis partner repeatedly talked down to you or shushed you.

You might be outraged because you're driving on the interstate, and you see a car in front of you litter for the second time in five minutes.

You might be full of hostility for 1001 reasons.

Or you might be full of rage because your hormones are unbalanced.

Ladies... We are allowed to be angry. Don't forget that. If you think your rage is because of your hormones, it probably is.

Moving on to tinnitus or ringing of the ears. I would argue that as you get older, your ears will ring a little bit more. For me, I wonder if it's hormonal? I think it's just one of the many joys of middle-age. I suppose it could be hormonal. But, I swear that if I concentrate on my ears, I hear a faint ringing sound.

Do you hear it too?!

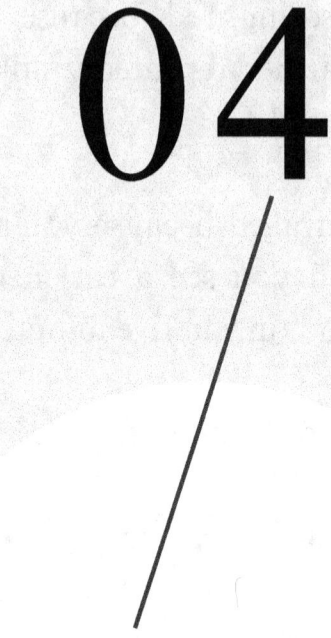

CHAPTER

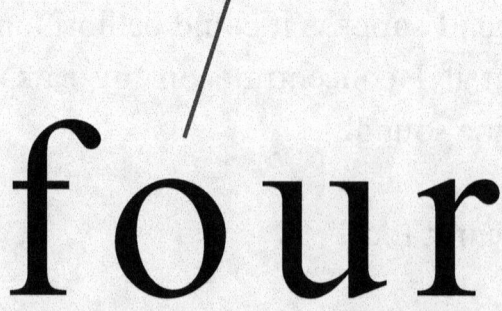

four

Chapter Four
Is the oven door open?

One autumn day, I was bringing my daughter's dirty laundry downstairs. Yes, she should've brought it down herself, but she was eight at the time - you pick your battles. I distinctly remember feeling like I was coming down with something because I felt the tiniest wave of warmth all over me. Maybe I was getting sick?

Unbeknownst to me, that was my first hot flash.

It happened a few more times before the lightbulb went off. During this time, my periods had been a little abnormal, but nothing that would cause concern. You know, a few days late or a few days early here and there. But these hot flashes were random and different. I don't know that I would even describe them as a hot flash, because I didn't sweat, and they were extremely mild. Think about walking outside from an air-conditioned room, for 1 to 2 seconds. That's what it felt like. And that's what it felt like for the next three years, maybe more.

I hope I'm describing to you just how minor these hot flashes were. They were barely noticeable. After the heart incident, I became highly in tune with my body. I started paying close attention. If my body wasn't in hyper-awareness mode, would I have even registered these as hot flashes? Who's to say?

Hot flashes... What exactly are they? And why do they happen?

Here's how I understand it. Our brain gets a faulty message saying, "I am overheating." This message triggers the body into cool-down mode. It's really the hypothalamus getting confused and rapid-firing messages throughout the body.

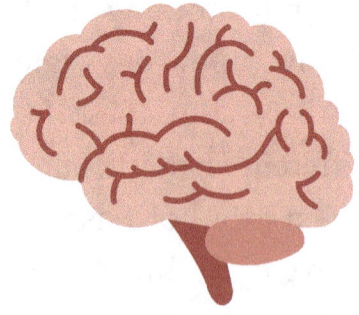

I'm better with visuals (see next page) when trying to explain the physiological and hormonal workings of the body.

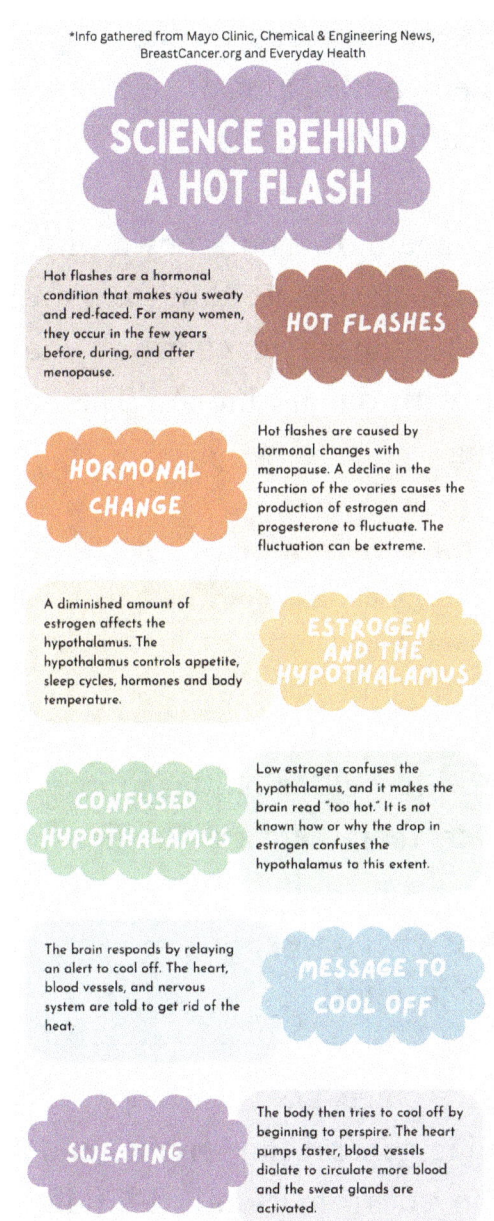

*Info gathered from Mayo Clinic, Chemical & Engineering News, BreastCancer.org and Everyday Health

SCIENCE BEHIND A HOT FLASH

Hot flashes are a hormonal condition that makes you sweaty and red-faced. For many women, they occur in the few years before, during, and after menopause.

HOT FLASHES

HORMONAL CHANGE

Hot flashes are caused by hormonal changes with menopause. A decline in the function of the ovaries causes the production of estrogen and progesterone to fluctuate. The fluctuation can be extreme.

A diminished amount of estrogen affects the hypothalamus. The hypothalamus controls appetite, sleep cycles, hormones and body temperature.

ESTROGEN AND THE HYPOTHALAMUS

CONFUSED HYPOTHALAMUS

Low estrogen confuses the hypothalamus, and it makes the brain read "too hot." It is not known how or why the drop in estrogen confuses the hypothalamus to this extent.

The brain responds by relaying an alert to cool off. The heart, blood vessels, and nervous system are told to get rid of the heat.

MESSAGE TO COOL OFF

SWEATING

The body then tries to cool off by beginning to perspire. The heart pumps faster, blood vessels dialate to circulate more blood and the sweat glands are activated.

So... Our hypothalamus gets confused? If that small part of the brain gets confused, what else is getting confused?

49

It is not known how or why the drop in estrogen confuses the hypothalamus to such an extent. Did you read that part?

Let's read it again. It is not known why...
There is so much that we don't know about Peri, including the inner workings of the brain in association with our hormones. The not knowing is frustrating.

Side note - Book II: The Meno Edition will talk more about the brain, theories about the relationship between the hypothalamus and estrogen, and how the pituitary gland is involved.

No wonder, I feel alone on this journey. There are fewer answers than there are questions.

Ladies... Are we screwed?
No. We are just hot!

○————————————○

Fast forward to age 45.
Remembering general time frames is difficult, but we had moved from South Florida to middle Georgia. Now, one would think that Florida would be hotter than Georgia, and it is, except for the summer.

This would've been my second Georgia summer. It was sometime in June, and it was unseasonably warm during the day, maybe 90°.

Our black lab, Indy, was outside, eating something she shouldn't be, so I had to fetch her. As I walked toward her, in an instant, my body felt like I had just opened up the oven door and hopped in.

I stopped in my tracks. I was shocked.

"What the fuck?" I said aloud.

Even Indy knew something was wrong because she quickly came to my side. Although I questioned what was happening, I knew exactly what it was.

"I hate you, Peri."

Great, now I'm talking to myself.

That was the first time I remember having a full-blown hot flash. It only lasted a few minutes. It started with my chest and radiated throughout my body. I broke out in a small sweat. I don't know that I would actually describe it as a sweat, it was more like my body instantly got clammy.

It was like a bizarre, out-of-body experience.

From that day on, hot flashes became my new normal. Some days I lost count. Some days I only had one. Research has shown that there are some triggers including, alcohol, spicy foods, stress, smoking, and wearing tight clothes. The only one that's obvious to me is spicy food. Spicy food is like throwing kerosene on a partially lit fire.

Don't get too freaked out. Some things can help...
A cold glass of water or an even colder beer works. Some say alcohol increases the odds of having a hot flash. I have not found that to be the case.

A neck fan. Surprisingly, it works wonders.

My personal favorite – opening up the freezer and standing in front of it.

My sister-in-law sent me a link to the most amazing product. It's a cooling mat for dogs. They recommend slipping in under your sheets for a cooler bed. Yes, please!

In the wintertime, our home stays pretty cool, because of Georgia's moderate weather. The summertime is brutal, and our AC pays the price.

Let's talk about night sweats! I've spoken to a lot of women. With the majority of those women, it seems like you either have random hot flashes throughout the day or whole-body, soaking night sweats. I am lucky enough to not have those wake-up-drenched, wash-the-sheets nights. Not yet.

I have so many Perimenopause symptoms. Life sometimes gives you small favors. No night sweats are one of them!

My experiences with hot flashes have been pretty consistent. They come and go. Winter helps. Summer sucks. Some weeks are worse than others. As I inch closer to Menopause, the hot flashes are intense, but I'm getting them less often.
Thank goodness.

Is there anything else that can be done to minimize or stop hot flashes and night sweats?

I found a great reference from menopausecenter.org:

Can You Ease Hot Flashes Naturally?

Absolutely. There are many natural ingredients that have been studied and identified as herbs that help minimize hot flashes. Look for dietary supplements that contain the ingredients below.

Key Ingredients to Help Alleviate Hot Flashes:
- Black Cohosh – This herb, derived from a species of buttercup, has proven safe and effective at reducing hot flashes and night sweats.

*Important side note - Before you start any kind of natural supplement for Peri, consult your doctor. It's important to understand drug interactions. For example, Black cohosh has the potential to interact with blood thinners and antiplatelet medications. The combination can risk the chance of bleeding.

- Red Clover – As a natural source of phytoestrogens called isoflavones, red clover is one herb that many women reach for when dealing with hot flashes.

- Soy – Soy contains isoflavones, which are plant estrogens. Some studies indicate that soy can be effective in reducing hot flashes.

- St. John's Wort – SJW is an herb that is known for having a calming effect on the nervous system. Many women claim that it also calms hot flashes.

Can You Prevent Hot Flashes?

While it's not always possible to prevent hot flashes, here are a few lifestyle changes that may help:

- Add a top-quality menopause supplement to your daily diet. *Your OB-GYN can offer recommendations.*
- Introduce clinically proven ingredients into your diet e.g. Black cohosh, Red Clover, and others such as Evening Primrose oil, Licorice root, Dong Quai, and Hibiscus. *Remember to always check with your doctor before adding a new supplement to your pill pad.*
- Stay hydrated.
- Cut out caffeine & alcohol *Not going to happen, Peri!*
- Dress in cotton or linen, cool, flowy clothing *Yesss! Let my inner boho queen shine.*
- Practice yoga & meditation.
- Don't exercise in the heat.
- Avoid spicy food.
- Maintain a cool room temperature.
  https://menopausecenter.org/menopause-info/

There are tons of supplements for Peri and Meno. Recently, I've tried Nature's Craft Menopause Support. It's packed full of herbs and vitamins mentioned in this chapter. I have to admit, I feel a bit better. Could be the placebo effect? Although I haven't tried it, I have a close friend who swears by bee pollen for her night sweats. She called it, "life-changing." Do me a favor, though? Chat with your Gyno before adding any supplements. They can help you find the right blend.

Trust them and remember that you can't always trust user reviews!

One night, in what seemed to be a hot flash peak, my hubby and I were watching an episode of "Suits," and I felt a big hot flash coming. And no, it wasn't from Harvey Specter.

I don't know why but I immediately pointed out my hot flash to my husband. I pulled down my shirt, exposing my chest, and said, "Feel this!"

His mind, of course, was in the gutter and he gave me a look like, "Really? (wink, wink)

"No - not that (low libido - another chapter). Get your mind out of the gutter. I want you to feel my hot flash."

I placed his hand in the middle of my chest.

"Gross. You are hot and sweaty."

Side note - Now husbands/partners... when we share something with you, physically, that may be gross, we would like you to react with curiosity, rather than disgust. Think, boys, think before you speak!

"No shit," I responded with annoyance. "How crazy is that?!

He wasn't as fascinated as I was. And just like that, the hot flash was gone. Back to Harvey Specter. Will you get with Donna, already?

To end this chapter, let's hear from some Reddit users describing a hot flash or night sweat.

"I describe my daytime hot flashes as being wrapped in a warm sheet after it comes out of the dryer. I've only had a few where it's break out full on sweat during the day." -Catnapbook

"I found it was much more difficult for my body to regulate its temperature in general leading up to menopause. So, if the day's temperature shifted, my body didn't respond in a timely fashion. Which would leave me overly hot or overly cold. Sometimes I'd feel like an oven, but no sweating, just radiating heat all over, sometimes I'd be teeth chattering cold on a balmy day. And in very warm temps my forearms would sweat heavily."
-Ragginghappy

"I get a swathe of heat from the neck outwards like a tidal wave, which lasts 2-3 minutes then dissipates over the next 5 mins, normally at night. My friend's face goes bright red & she starts sweating like a fountain & her hair starts to drip, any time of day or night." -Tillymint54

"I get hot but it's mostly internal but sometimes my neck and chest get warm. I don't sweat. It feels like I'm vibrating internally too." -Anne-Hedonia9

"My hot flashes are more like I wake up in sweat. I don't actually feel myself getting hot (because I'm sleeping) I just wake up and my hair is wet, my t-shirt neck is wet and sometimes the pillowcase is a bit damp. I also usually have sweat on my chest." -Onlykitten

"When I've had hot flashes during the day they're more intense-like this heat comes from inside me and pretty quickly I'm sweating (usually again head, neck and chest). Sometimes I even feel a bit sick to my stomach - that's rare - but it passes very quickly." -Onlykitten

"I feel like I'm glowing fiercely for a short amount of time and very infrequently. Have more in the way of night sweats which are a bit of a pain." -Unlucky_Fan_6079

"When they are really bad it's like a panic attack. It feels like I'm suffocating from my own body heat. My face feels like it's on fire and then it spreads to the rest of my body and I need to cool off. I've been using Meno supplements. They aren't as bad now but still a nuisance at night." -PaleDifference

"It was like a core of lava would flare up inside of me. I would start to sweat and feel trapped, it happens very quickly, something like 30 seconds from normal to dying." -Tinycowz

"Before I started on HRT, they were mainly night sweats. I'd wake in the night with my heart thumping, feeling sick, sweaty and like I had hypoglycemia. During the day I would just have swamp crotch! Now I'm on HRT, it's a lot better, I struggle occasionally with temperature regulation, but it passes pretty quickly." -Marestar13134

"For me (this is me speaking), it's like that feeling when you first walk into a sauna. It's also like opening up an oven. and the heat washes over you. I sweat under my boobs and at the nape of my neck. When I play tennis and have a hot flash, I get overheated and lightheaded, and my entire body breaks a sweat. Mine last 3-5 minutes, at most." -Angie Schwendeman

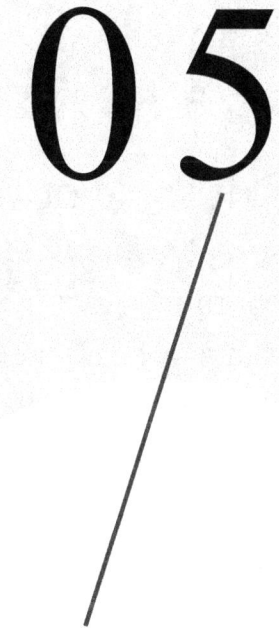

05

CHAPTER

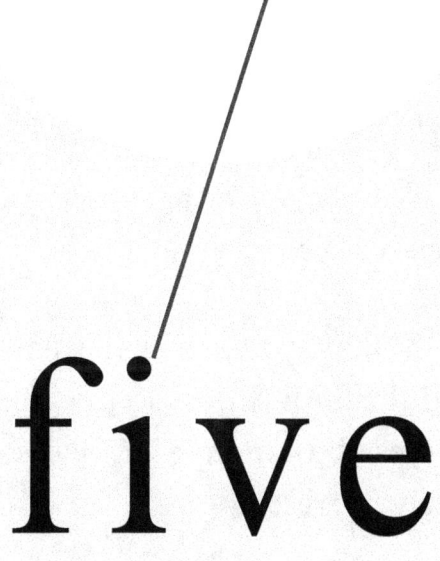

five

Chapter Five
Did I just become a bleeder?

There was just SO MUCH BLOOD.

It's embarrassing. I know from personal experience. I'm no stranger to a heavy period. The only time I didn't have a heavy period was during the brief time that I was on the pill (and of course, when I was prego).

This takes me back to high school. The memory is so vivid. I can remember the bathroom stall... I can remember that small, geometric, dirty tile floor. I can remember my thighs covered in red. It was between classes, so the bathroom was busy, and I only had a couple of minutes. I was running to the stall because I could feel the blood gushing.

Side note- I know that you know THAT feeling. This was in the beginning of my menstrual journey before I wore tampons. I was basically wearing a diaper. I remember the sound that it made while walking. I always wondered if I was the only one that could hear it?

Where was I? Okay, so I ran to the stall, closed the door, locked the door, lifted up my green and blue plaid skirt (yes, I went to Catholic school), and was absolutely horrified.

There was just so much blood.
Panic set in. Where do I even begin? I need to get to class. Is there enough toilet paper? And the smell... I remember that too. I'm sure I don't need to tell you this, but I was late for class because, cleanup on aisle 7, took F O R E V E R.

From that day forward, I tried to be creative during the heaviest times of my menstrual cycle. I had pads stashed everywhere. I had them in my locker, in every pocket of my backpack, in my tennis bag, in my jacket pockets. You get my drift. I tried different things... wearing two super duper pads. That didn't work, too bulky. I tried wearing one pad and wading up tons of toilet paper on top, for extra coverage. That worked a little bit. I had backup clothes. I had backups for my backups. I had a cardigan whose sole purpose was to tie around my waist. It was the 90s, after all.

All of that, and I talked to no one about it.
I still can't figure out why that is? I guess, I was young and embarrassed. There was a family mentality of "suck it up" and "stick your head in the sand." Looking back - that was the wrong way to live.

Thank goodness for one of the girls on the tennis team. She was a senior, and she took me under her wing.

Side note- Of course, in tennis we wore white skirts. So stupid. I get it (sort of). Tennis...Wimbledon...wear your tennis whites...but let's change that! For those non-tennis players out there, at Wimbledon, there is an all-white dress code for players.
Before you get angry at the traditions of tennis in England, in a change announced late last year, female players now have the option of wearing dark-colored undershorts, provided they are no longer than their shorts or skirt. It's a start.

My new favorite senior asked me if I needed a tampon. She was in the toilet next to me. I am guessing she knew I was on my period and struggling. In my utter embarrassment, I said yes. From under the stall, she passed me a Super Tampax *(SUPER)*. I came face-to-face with my fear and stuck that thing in me. I will never forget her or her small kindness. Life after that got a lot easier.

And that's just an example of high school heavy bleeding! There is definitely a correlation between heavy high school bleeding and heavy Peri bleeding. You guessed it... Fluctuating hormones.

Perimenopause bleeding is heavy and random. This is not the case for everyone. It was certainly the case for me. Like I said before, I am no stranger to heavy periods. I've considered my periods heavy for most of my life. This is a different type of heavy. It's heavy, by way of clots.

Blood clots can be alarming, and they are something that you should always bring up to your doctor. They can also be very normal during Peri.

Halfway through my Peri journey, I remember having an extra heavy period. On day two, I could hardly wear a tampon because the giant blood clots were pushing it out. By giant, I mean the size of a medium-sized strawberry. Now, I know that's gross, but I'm not here to sugarcoat things. I wish I had known that these large, quarter-size, and bigger clots were going to happen.

Let's go to the science of it. A menstrual clot is a mix of blood and tissue released from the uterus during a period. They are characterized by jelly-like globules and unusually thick blood. Women can consider clotting as the body's natural way of protecting itself. Those clots prevent too much blood from leaving the body at one time.

Small clots, the size of a nickel and smaller are normal. The size of the clot matters a lot more than the color.

I am laughing out loud at this next part because my Peri and Meno research shows that I was actually suffering from menorrhagia (The medical term for periods with unusually heavy bleeding).

Monitor Other Symptoms to Verify...
Women who suspect menorrhagia may also suffer from other abnormalities, aside from unusual period clots, including:

- Soaking through a pad or tampon every hour for several hours ✓
- Symptoms of anemia, like fatigue and tiredness ✓
- Limiting daily activities because of heavy flow ✓
- Waking up during the night to change sanitary protection ✓
- Using double protection to catch all the blood ✓
- Period lasting longer than a week ✓

Having any of these symptoms necessitates seeking medical help promptly before further complications arise.

https://www.medicalnewstoday.com/articles/295202

My bleeding was so erratic. Some periods were barely there. I would have spotting between periods, and sometimes in the place of a normal period. The last two years of my cycle were bizarre, with a mixture of skipped periods and gushers. There wasn't a lot of rhyme and reason to it. My hormones were in control. I was not.

I wasn't able to find any science to back up this claim, but I had a crazy experience with giving blood. I really think it's Peri-related. The last two times I had blood drawn, once I was bandaged up, I sprouted a significant leak. The first time it happened, the nurse said, "Oh! You are a bleeder."

"I am?!" I asked in horror, as the blood was gushing down my arm.

From then on, I made sure to mention to the person taking my blood, that *I am a bleeder.*

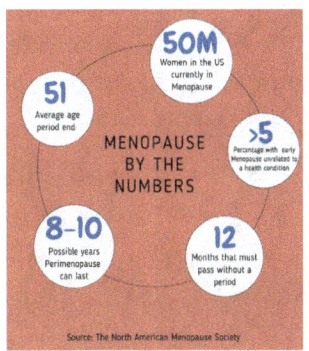

MENOPAUSE BY THE NUMBERS

5OM Women in the US currently in Menopause

51 Average age period end

>5 Percentage with early Menopause unrelated to a health condition

8-10 Possible years Perimenopause can last

12 Months that must pass without a period

Source: The North American Menopause Society

Like I said before, ladies, this journey of Peri and Meno was a huge learning experience. I found myself down some random and dark rabbit holes, in my search of Peri knowledge. I also found a couple of articles that were so spectacular. I found one in particular that I am going to add larger snippets of it. It was that good.

There will be blood: women on the shocking truth about periods and perimenopause - by Gabi Hinsliff

If Emma Pickett needs to make a long journey, she checks her calendar very carefully. She will often take an emergency change of clothes when she goes out, and if giving a lecture for work, has to ensure it is no longer than half an hour. Yet she rarely hears anyone talk about the reason so many older women secretly go to all this trouble; why they've started to stick to black trousers, give up the sports they loved, or plan days out – especially with children – meticulously.

"If you have a bunch of 12-year-olds in the car, you can't say: 'Sorry chaps, I'm just bleeding heavily today,'" says Pickett, a 48-year-old breastfeeding counselor and author of The Breast Book, who also happens to be among the one in five British women who suffer from heavy periods in the run-up to menopause (or perimenopause). "You can talk about hot flushes, make a joke about it. But because menstrual blood is gross in our society, there's no conversation about it. There must be women round the world just pretending they need to dash off for some other reason."

Michelle Obama has spoken frankly about coping with hot flushes (the Brits call them *flushes*) in the White House, and the Countess of Wessex recently confessed to having suffered menopausal brain fog. But it takes a different level of courage to talk publicly about wearing three pairs of knickers – just in case, or to cope with what the Canadian gynecologist and author of "The Menopause Manifesto" Dr Jen Gunter calls a "supersoaker event" – the kind of bleeding that can flood through clothes, defeat even a combination of super-plus tampons and maternity towels, and leave women needing iron supplements or in some cases stop them leaving the house.

Some remain reluctant to seek treatment for what Nicola, 52, still considers "an inconvenience rather than an illness", despite being forced to sit on blankets to protect her sofa. But others describe battling with unsympathetic doctors. "I often see people who have been left to feel there wasn't anything to be done," says Gunter, whose book includes an entire chapter on midlife periods aimed at demystifying the problem. "But no one ever says erectile dysfunction is 'just a part of men's lives', do they? We can say this is a typical thing that happens – and there's treatment if you want it."

"Carolyn Harris, the Labour MP and chair of the all-party parliamentary group on menopause, was 50 when she finally saw her doctor about the heavy periods she had suffered for years. "I'd be sitting in a chair and as long as I was sitting down, I was fine, but when I got up it was, literally, a gush and I'd just be absolutely saturated," says Harris, who was working as an MP's assistant.

https://www.theguardian.com/society/2021/jul/22/there-will-be-blood-women-on-the-shocking-truth-about-periods-and-perimenopause

Can anything be done for Peri's heavy bleeding or heavy bleeding in general? Yes, of course! I made the mistake of thinking my heavy bleeding was normal. Looking back, I don't believe it was. Remedies range from all-natural and non-hormonal, to hormonal and surgical.

HOW TO REMEDY
Heavy Periods

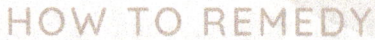

NATURAL

Use ice packs - placing an ice pack on the abdomen several times a day may reduce blood flow.
Aromatherapy - cypress, geranium and rose are claimed effective for reducing blood flow.
Eat iron rich foods.
Supplement with vitamins - Vitamin C helps the body absorb iron. Vitamin A, E, B, and K are also credited for helping slow menstrual flow.
Drink raspberry infusion - Herbalists say drinking a daily infusion of raspberry leaf helps the uterus and ovaries slow heavy bleeding.
Exercise and meditate regularly.
Consider acupuncture.

NON-HORMONAL

Ibuprofen can help with heavy bleeding by reducing the amount of your flow.
Prescription-only anti-inflammatory painkillers with naproxen can help with heavy bleeding.
Tranexamic acid is a non-hormonal prescription drug used to treat heavy menstrual bleeding.

HORMONAL

Hormonal IUDs release progestin and help control heavy bleeding.
Oral progesterone or a progestin. Prescribed progesterone is also manufactured in a lab and is molecularly identical to the progesterone made in our bodies. Progestins have a different molecular structure. Progestins are stronger than natural progesterone and are said to be better for controlling heavy menstrual bleeding.
Combined or progestin only birth control pills.

SURGICAL

Endometrial ablation or resection where the lining of the uterus is surgically destroyed or removed to slow or stop menstrual flow.
Hysterectomy which is the removal of the uterus.
If polyps or fibroids are found to be causing your heavy bleeding, surgical removal of these tissues may be recommended.

https://www.menopausenow.com/irregular-periods/articles/how-to-stop-heavy-periods-10-natural-remedies
https://thisisperimenopause.com/symptoms/heavy-bleeding-in-perimenopause/

Whether you are in Peri, Meno, or just a woman with "normal periods," I think it's safe to say that we've all been there. Not many chat about it and that needs to change. We need to normalize talking about it, amongst ourselves, with our doctors, with spouses, and even with employers. Yes, it's not an easy subject to bring up. But is that a good enough reason?

Are we supposed to suffer in silence? To hell with that! I refuse. Peri is a fickle bitch and she's different for everyone. Discuss the best options with your doctor. Advocate for yourselves. Do your research. Don't let Peri rain on your parade.

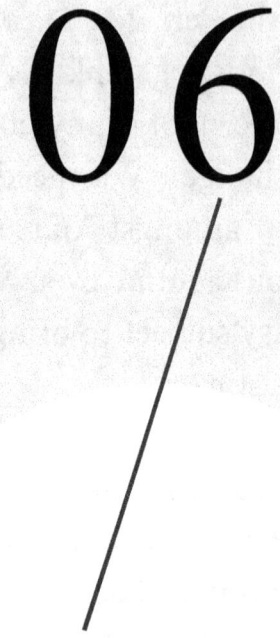

06

CHAPTER

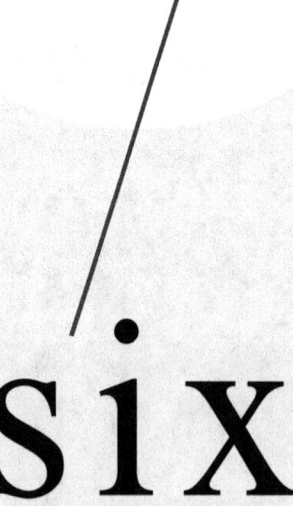

six

Chapter Six
WTF is going on with my face?

"Alexa, is grapefruit good for your skin?"
If Alexa could talk, she would say, "Yes, Angie, but collagen is better."
But she can't, and her response was, "Because grapefruit is rich in vitamin C, and vitamin A, consuming grapefruit or grapefruit juice will help nourish your skin."

As I sit here, eating my grapefruit, hoping it's the fountain of youth, I can only tell you that the skin changes are not fun. The changes are gradually sudden. Between the weight gain (we will get to that in a few chapters) and the skin changes, I don't feel like myself.

At first, I thought it was the products that I was using, new and old. But new products shouldn't cause sunspots, should they? I was experiencing a mixture of acne, sunspots, wrinkles, and sagging skin.
"What the fuck is going on with my face?!" I said to my girl, Indy. She tilted her head as if to say, "Don't ask me?"

Let's rewind.

For decades, I made the mistake of thinking that the sun was my friend. It made me feel good. I have an olive skin tone, so I would tan beautifully. My confidence would skyrocket as my skin got more and more bronzed. Yes, I was a teenager in the 90s. Along with the thin eyebrows, I frequented the tanning bed.

Hindsight is 20/20, I know, but that was dumb. Like many younger girls, I was indeed an idiot. My skin and eyebrows are now paying the price.

Side note – Spring break is coming up and I'm taking my daughter to Daytona Beach. Yesterday, she asked me to take her to Target to pick up some products. Here I was thinking to myself, yay! I've taught her well. She's seen my face and wants to take care of her face. It was such a proud moment, until we got there, and she went straight for the no SPF bronzing tanning oil.
Touché, karma.

Growing up, I was extremely fortunate because in those formative teenage years, I had little to no acne. I treated my skin like shit. I didn't wear much make up, but when I did, I slept in it.

Between the occasional use of Noxzema, and let's not forget about St. Ives Apricot Scrub (on my face!!!), I had no real skincare routine.

My daughter is 14. She and I are like two hormonal ships passing in the night. I will say, her skin is flawless. Her vanity is covered with Sephora products. As much as I shake my head at the amount of money she spends on beauty products, she doesn't realize it now, but she is helping the longevity of her skin. But she doesn't want to wear sunscreen?! One battle at a time. Am I right?

Back to my own battles... The first thing I noticed with Peri was my hormonal acne. Most of my acne was small. They were tiny whiteheads and blemishes on my lower cheeks and chin. My acne was extremely minor, hardly noticeable to anyone but me. I tried pimple patches (that I stole from my daughter). They didn't work. I tried covering it up with makeup, and I really think that made it worse. I also made the ginormous mistake of buying one of those 10X mirrors. If you really want to feel unattractive, do that!

Side note - Who am I kidding? I need the 20X mirror to pluck the eyebrows and chin hair. See Chapters 13 and 17.

My husband, for my birthday, bought some expensive skin "elixir." I've been diligently using it, but I can't tell the difference. It's so hard to know what products are the right products. Next stop, the dermatologist.

Side note - I went to the Dermatologist, and they gave me Retin-A (Tretinoin). IT'S WORKING and my blemishes are disappearing!

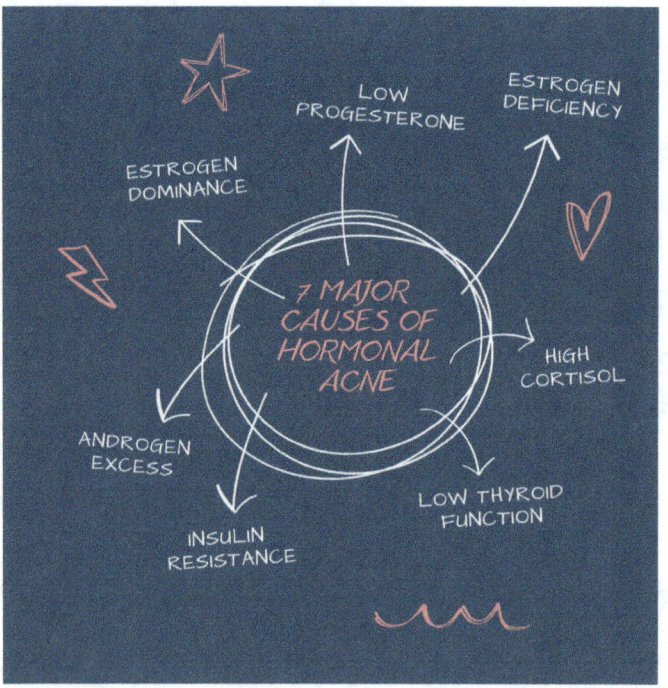

Peri causes acne mostly due to decreased estrogen and stress. But those aren't the only culprits.

Here are pieces of an article from Byrdie.com, "How to Treat Menopausal Acne, According to Dermatologists,"

Levels of estrogen, the so-called female hormone, plummet rapidly during Peri/Meno, throwing off the delicate balance of androgens, most specifically testosterone. "As estrogen levels fall, the relative increase of testosterone results in oily skin and clogged pores," explains Cheung. That spike of testosterone also causes increased facial hair growth and is why this type of acne shows up on the lower face. As it seems that this is where more androgen receptors live.

They continue to chat about stress.

Any woman who has experienced or is experiencing Meno will quickly tell you, it's a stressful time. Unfortunately, this becomes a double-edged sword: "Stress due to the many other changes happening within the body also contributes to acne," Rodney says. Along with impacting hormone levels in general, stress increases cortisol in the body, the aptly dubbed stress hormone. "It wreaks havoc on the skin in many ways, triggering breakouts through increased oil production being just one of them," she says. While it's obviously easier said than done, attempting to reduce stress, as much as possible, during, before, and after Menopause is paramount.

https://www.byrdie.com/menopausal-acne-5114119

So, let me get this straight...

I'm stressed because my face is breaking out, like never before. The stress combined with the higher levels of testosterone and the lower levels of estrogen, makes me not only get pimples, but it also causes a list of other things?

Lovely.

The article goes on to say that the best remedy is from the inside out.

Fix the hormones - fix the acne
Fix the stress - fix the acne

If it were only that simple.

Let's keep being real. It's not just acne that is the problem. Ladies, it gets worse. I started with some minor hormonal skin issues.
The next issue is more concerning (to me), because I'm currently going through it. At first, I thought it was melasma, but it is turned out to be just sun/age spots.

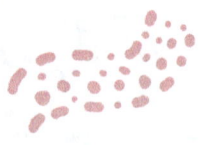

Both are cosmetic issues that surround Peri.

Not only is she a bitch, she's also a speckled bitch.

If you are anything like me, you may be wondering what the differences are between age spots and melasma? Both are forms of hyperpigmentation.

Melasma is a skin condition that causes dark patches on the skin, usually on the face. It is caused by a combination of hormonal changes and sun exposure. In their 40s and 50s, as women enter Peri, estrogen production decreases, allowing testosterone to become the dominant hormone in their bodies. This triggers melanin production, along with hair growth and sometimes oilier skin. The hormonal fluctuation you get in Peri could also cause higher estrogen levels, alternating with low levels, and could also contribute to melasma.

Your hormones are constantly changing during Peri. Up, down, up down. Those huge fluctuations make it very difficult to test for hormonal deficiencies. You would practically have to test hormones daily, in order to get an accurate assessment.

When these different hormones become unbalanced, it causes the body to literally go berserk! This is not the case for everyone, but my body certainly did.

As of right now, my age spots are more prevalent. It's like I turned into a Dalmatian overnight.
Again - my carefree, sun-loving past is biting me in my pale ass... (except that one fine day, on a deserted beach in the south of France).

Sunspots, also called age spots, and "liver spots" (even though they have absolutely nothing to do with the liver) are hyperpigmented skin blemishes. They are small, flat, dark spaces on the skin. Shocker! They are caused by the sun. Melanin can build up on areas of the skin that have gotten too much sun over the years.

Difference between melasma, sunspots, and freckles?
The biggest difference is in the shape. Melasma is blotchy and large in size. Think about a shadow on parts of your face. Freckles are small, round spots with clear edges, and they are hereditary. Sunspots look like freckles, but they are asymmetrical. Sunspots are also larger than freckles.

The causes of melasma are mostly hormonal changes and sun exposure. Freckles are caused by genetics and sun exposure. Sunspots are caused by age and sun exposure.

All right, so I got too much sun, spent too much time in tanning beds, etc. What does this have to do with Peri? Well, it mostly boils down to estrogen. Estrogen helps control melanin production. Melanin is the pigment in your skin, eyes, and hair. So, as you can imagine, if estrogen levels decrease, then melanin production increases. This leads to age spots.

That's part one...

Taking a small break to add sunscreen to my Amazon cart.

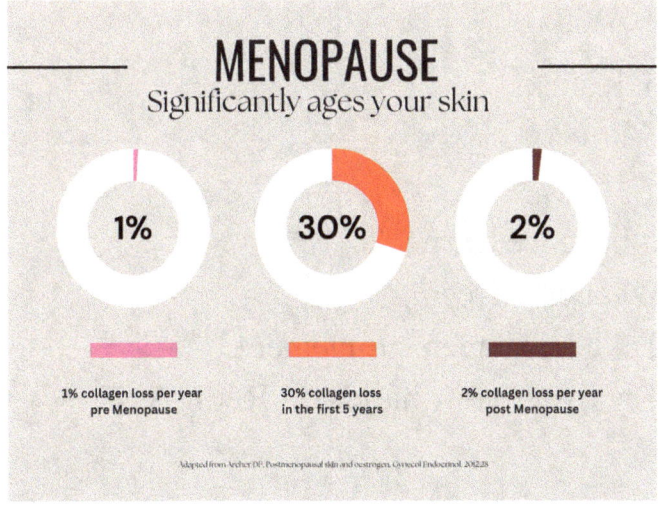

MENOPAUSE
Significantly ages your skin

1%

30%

2%

1% collagen loss per year
pre Menopause

30% collagen loss
in the first 5 years

2% collagen loss per year
post Menopause

Adapted from Archer DF. Postmenopausal skin and oestrogen. Gynecol Endocrinol. 2012;28

We've covered estrogen and melanin. Now let's dive into collagen. Collagen is a protein that is the primary building block of skin and other connective tissue. It's responsible for healthy joints and skin elasticity.

Collagen production slows down as we age. During Peri and Meno, we know that estrogen drops dramatically. The drop in estrogen can reduce the body's ability to synthesize collagen. If our estrogen levels are dropping, our collagen levels are also dropping. All of a sudden, our skin loses elasticity, wrinkles, and fine lines form.

I've noticed some sagging skin in my eyelids, under my eyes, and in my jowls. Oh, and I almost forgot… the neck wrinkles!

Yeah, it sucks.

What have we learned?
1. Wear sunscreen.
2. Take a collagen supplement.
3. Try to get your hands on Retin-A.

What else can be done? Well, that's up to you. There are thousands of at-home remedies. Do you have lemon juice or apple cider vinegar in your pantry/fridge? They are both natural skin brighteners and can help hyperpigmentation. Do they work? I suppose that depends on the person.

Talk with your doctor, dermatologist, or Ob-gyn. Come up with a game plan. Don't be like me... Be proactive instead of reactive. I thought for the longest time that I wanted to age naturally. I can still do that. And I will, but there are things, natural things that can be done to combat the brutality of Peri.

For me, I wear more sunscreen than ever before. I should do it more often, but I do take collagen supplements. Note to self – do that every day. My Peri diet consists of more skin and anti-inflammatory foods. I try to drink a ton of water. I have one of those at home, red-light therapy wands. I've tried a lot of the trendy masks, but I don't think they work.
They can't hurt, right?

Here is my hard truth, I don't feel like myself. I don't look like myself, and that is heartbreaking at times. I'm going to be very honest and vulnerable with you... Peri has made me feel unattractive. Five to 10 years ago, I used to say,

"I'll die with these wrinkles."

Now, I think differently. I haven't gone down the Botox route, yet, but for the first time in my life, I am thinking about it. Looking in the mirror can be tough. I feel old. I feel weathered. I feel spotty. Some days, I feel fat. Most days, I don't feel pretty.

Okay, okay. Enough of the pity party!

My long-winded point... You are not alone. Just because people don't talk about it, doesn't mean they don't feel it. We are beautiful. Our wrinkles are a sign that we lived, laughed, and loved. Let's have our age spots serve as a youthful memory of topless (and bottomless) beaches and adventure. I am constantly reminding myself that Peri is volatile, but I'm stronger than she will ever be.

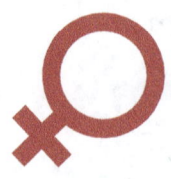

That being said, I need to be better at taking care of my skin (and myself). As a mom, sometimes I put my needs last. We do that, don't we? It's so easy to be self-sacrificial. I, for one, can tell you that my skin is suffering! So, take care of yourselves, ladies! Get that facial that you've always wanted to get. Splurge on better moisturizer with SPF. Go to the dermatologist annually and be honest with them. If you want to see a change in your skin, they can make that happen. Don't be afraid to take care of you.

And don't forget... Wear sunscreen!

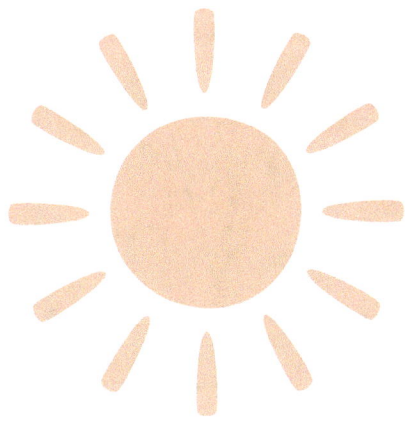

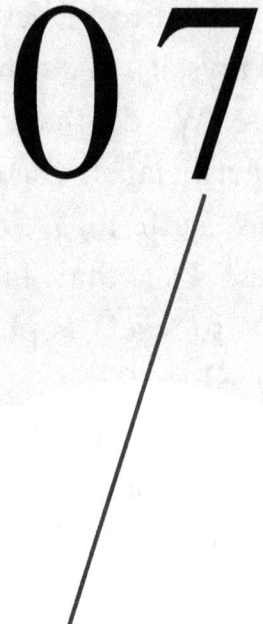

07

CHAPTER

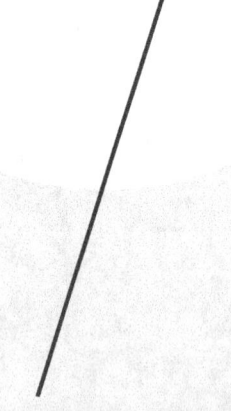

seven

Chapter Seven
Did I just pee myself?

Yes. Yes, I did.

Now, you can imagine my absolute surprise and horror, the first, second, third, fourth, fifth, and tenth time this happened.
I was mortified and embarrassed. Thank goodness it happened at home.

I can remember it like it was yesterday. I was outside playing soccer with my daughter. This was about four years ago, so she was 10 years old, and I was 43.
I was trying to defend, and my daughter made a sick move around me. For all of you soccer fans, she successfully did the Maradona. I laughed. It wasn't a comical laugh; it was a proud laugh. It was a laugh that was accompanied by the internal monologue of,
"That little shit (proud mom moment) just passed me."

The laugh was also accompanied by a sprint to catch up to her.

That. Was. All. It. Took.

"Did I just pee myself?"
I knew the answer.
I wasn't ready to announce it to the world and my daughter, so I just very discreetly excused myself.
The potty confirmed what I already knew. It was just a couple of drops, but it was enough to make me question everything.
Leading up to this, I had heard the stories, heard the whispers. Urine leakage.

The bright green visual of a package of Depends immediately popped into my mind.
"It can't be. I'm too young for this."
That sentence needs to be banned from my vernacular. At that point, I did a panicked Google search.

I typed... I am 43. Why did my bladder just leak?

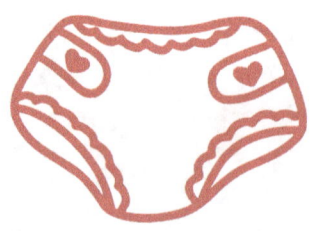

Yes, I took a screenshot!

🔒 Q i'm 43, why did — Private

MORE RESULTS

Does menopause make you pee yourself? ⌄

Why does my bladder leak in my 40s? ⌃

Pregnancy, childbirth, hormonal changes associated with the menopause and putting 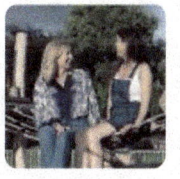 on weight are some of the many causes of bladder leakage due to weakening pelvic floor muscles. These issues are more commonly experienced by older women, but it can just as easily affect someone in their 30s or even younger. Sep 5, 2019

N https://www.news-medical.net › news

Two-thirds of women over 40 suffer from bladder leakage, research ...

MORE RESULTS

The next few months, and even years, turned into the ultimate science project. What would cause the leakage? Could I prevent it? Will it get worse?

Enter Kegel exercises.

Do they help? Hell yes, they do. But you have to be diligent with them (which I am not). Remember me, reactive, not proactive. Proactive? More like prolapse.

Two-thirds of women over 40 suffer from bladder leakage! Two-freaking-thirds!!!

I bet you can guess why? Stupid hormones.

Side note- I have taught my daughter to find another word other than stupid. Fine. Asinine. Hormones are asinine.

Broken record, but when you're in your Peri stage, estrogen levels decrease. This drop in hormones causes urogenital tissues to become stiffer and thinner, weakening your pelvic floor muscles. Because pelvic floor weakness naturally occurs as you age, women experiencing Peri are more likely to leak urine during this time.

I'm afraid to tell you this, but it got worse from there. It started happening more and more with activity.

All kinds of activity, wink, wink.

No, I told myself that I was going to be brutally honest in this book. Sex made me leak (I'm sorry, daughter, if you ever read this). Talk about mortifying?! The good news is, my husband was oblivious. Nonetheless, I was so embarrassed.

Enter Kegel exercises, again.

Sometimes, I need these embarrassing reminders to do the things that I know I should be doing regularly. Strengthen that pelvic floor!

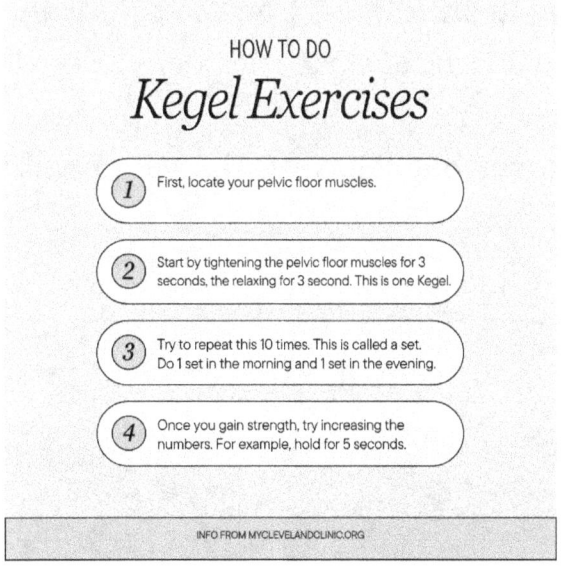

HOW TO DO
Kegel Exercises

1. First, locate your pelvic floor muscles.

2. Start by tightening the pelvic floor muscles for 3 seconds, the relaxing for 3 second. This is one Kegel.

3. Try to repeat this 10 times. This is called a set. Do 1 set in the morning and 1 set in the evening.

4. Once you gain strength, try increasing the numbers. For example, hold for 5 seconds.

INFO FROM MYCLEVELANDCLINIC.ORG

So... My scientific experiment, over the next few years, came up with the following conclusive evidence:

I can run. I can laugh. But I can't run and laugh at the same time.

There is a general urgency to go, one that I didnt have before.

I can sneeze. But if I sneeze hard, I'm crossing my legs, because it could go either way. If you ever see a woman in the grocery store who sneezes and crosses her legs at the same time, now you know why.

I can play tennis. But if I hit the ball really hard or go for an overhead smash, leak city.

I can laugh, but I have to be very careful about belly laughing.

I can now no longer make fun of my mother for getting up in the middle of the night to urinate. I am that girl now.

I haven't thrown up in a long time, but I imagine THAT amount of force would cause a urinary blowout.

Kegels help. Period undies help more.

Baths hinder. I love my baths, especially with Epsom salt, but they cause more leakage.

Sex is hit or miss.

I made the mistake of jumping on a trampoline, once, in my 40s. This is wrong on so many levels. But yes, it caused me to dribble. I have to laugh about it. Don't laugh too hard!

I sincerely hope I'm not exaggerating this new "condition." It doesn't happen often. When it does happen, it's always during something physical. It didn't take me long to figure out exactly when it would happen.

Tennis is the biggest culprit. But I know that going in, so when I play tennis, I am overly prepared. I have several pairs of period underwear. I always get the heaviest flow possible, simply because I tried the "slim to regular flow," and those were a joke. They weren't catching anything.

Also, the color black is your friend. Quick dry material is your friend. Black and quick-dry, and you are safe for days. I made the mistake, once, of wearing the light-flow undies with gray bottoms. I should've known better. I rarely wear gray tops, because of how well they show sweat, what would possess me to think that I could get away with sporting gray capris?

I don't think anyone noticed. I noticed! I've learned that people, especially when you're playing sports, don't look at your crotch.
Surprising, right?
Either way, it was a live-and-learn moment. I only wear black on the bottom. Better safe than sorry.

I've become a source of comic relief for my family. After I got a handle of the urine leakage, I confided in my family about it.
They were understanding, at first. Then, after a small amount of time passed, the inside jokes started rolling. My family (husband and daughter) think that they are quite the comedians.

On a serious note, I am glad I told my fam about it. In a crazy way, Peri has brought us together. We laugh a lot more (at me) because of the random side effects of her (Peri).

At first, their laughs made me angry. I don't think it was their laughs, per se. I think I was just angry that my body was malfunctioning. I think I was angry because, for the first time in my life, I was getting up in the middle of the night to pee. I think I was angry because I had to worry about my bladder leaking while doing normal things. I eventually got over it, but there was certainly an adjustment period.

I used to laugh at my friend, Amanda. That girl had the smallest bladder and had to pee so often. I never understood it because I was the opposite. I never had to pee. I could hold it until I got home. Until I couldn't.

Amanda – now I get it!

Let's chat a bit more about the physiology and science of it all.

I absolutely hate the word incontinence. I don't know why, but I feel like that word is shrouded in negativity and embarrassment. That's probably why I haven't used it. From a scientific perspective, I'm going to have to use the word here.

Some studies have shown that in your middle years, especially those around Peri and Meno, you're at increased risk of developing one or two types of urinary incontinence.
Going through Peri, and mostly Meno has been linked with stress incontinence. That's the first type.

Stress incontinence is mostly caused by weak, pelvic floor muscles. The most common symptoms are leaking urine while coughing, laughing, sneezing, or lifting heavy objects. This type of incontinence is common during Peri but typically doesn't worsen because of Meno. Hallelujah.

Side note - This is me! I try to not lift heavy objects, for what should be obvious reasons! One of the future chapters (Head, shoulders, knees, and toes) will discuss this.

The second type is urge incontinence. This commonly happens more in the later years. It's also called "overactive bladder." Urge incontinence is exactly like it sounds. You have the urge to pee a lot more often. It is the sudden and strong urge to urinate, which can result in a loss of bladder control before you reach the toilet. Also, waking up several times during the night to pee is another type of urge incontinence.

Side note - I do this - but it's usually only once, and it generally depends on how much water I drink after 8 pm. I don't know about you, but I tend to drink most of my water in the PM. The day gets away from me and by the time I get home and start to unwind, my lips are dry, and I think to myself, I should drink more water. So, I chug about 64oz. My body thanks me by waking up at 2 am, and maybe again at 5 am. You'd think I would learn. We will just blame this one on Peri. She's a great scapegoat.

Have no fear! I know these symptoms are scary, but for me, they are minor. For most, they are minor.
There are also treatments and different lifestyle changes that can help the pelvic floor.
Some women choose hormone therapy. I've talked to several women who say the same thing, I wish I would've taken hormones sooner.

There are also non-hormonal treatments for bladder control. These include:
Urinary supplements,

Reducing caffeine, *reducing maybe - giving up, never.*

Bladder training techniques that increase the capacity to hold urine,

Maintaining a healthy weight,

Avoiding stress to the pelvic area and doing Kegel exercises,

Electrical stimulation of the bladder muscles, a pessary device, inserted to help hold up a prolapsed bladder,

A device placed in the urethra, that blocks leakage,

Various surgical techniques to restructure support for the bladder.

But ladies, I will say this again…
Don't suffer in silence.
Talk with your doctor.

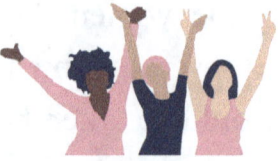

08

CHAPTER

eight

Chapter Eight
Do I need Weight Watchers?

You know how men get a "Dad bod?" I'm definitely getting a "Peri bod."

Do I need Weight Watchers? I feel like I do. I need something. This weight gain seemed to happen overnight.

Here's a little bit about me... I've never been a small person. I have an athletic build and wide hips. I'm 5'8" (used to be taller). If I weighed 165 pounds, that was amazing for me. My realistic goal now is to weigh 175 pounds. That equates to a size 10-12. Right now, I am a solid size 12 and 190 pounds. I don't love it. This is the biggest that I've ever been except for being pregnant. I gained a lot of weight during pregnancy but, I also had an almost 9-pound baby.

I'm a bit of a pear shape. I've always been a little thicker from my belly button and below. From my belly button and above, up until about five years ago, I was always pretty trim. Having a baby changes things, and it did change my body. I got a little bit wider, but I didn't change sizes. Things just started to fit a little differently.

That bitch, Peri, she doesn't like pears. She prefers apples. At least, that's the shape I'm turning into. I've never had a tiny waist. No hourglass shape for me, but like I said earlier, it was always pretty trim. Now, I feel like my waist is getting bigger and bigger.

I feel like my weight has shifted. My legs have gotten skinnier from playing tennis and pickleball, but my waist, stomach, boobs, hips have all gotten larger. My face has gained some weight as well.

I've tried dietary change. It seemed to help, minimally. I've tried not drinking. Again, minimal or no change. I cut out beer a long time ago and now solely drink red wine. Anyone who knows me can attest that I don't drink much, and I don't eat much.

Genetics plays a factor, of course. My family isn't full of really skinny people. Right now, I don't think it's a genetics thing. I think, like everything else in this book, it's a hormonal thing.

I noticed the weight gain in pictures. When I was in a friend's wedding, I couldn't help but see that my arms looked bigger. It was so obvious, to me. This was several years ago, in the thick of Peri.

So, in my mind, I'm doing a lot of the right things. I drink plenty of water. I try to limit the carbs and the alcohol. I exercise by playing tennis and pickleball, at a fairly competitive level, so I'm burning a lot of calories.

It's not working. At this point, I'm not gaining anymore, but I'm not losing. As vulnerable as this sounds, I feel fat. It's the truth, and I know I'm not alone in saying it.

This is the first time in my life that I don't like looking in the mirror. I've never been an overly confident person, but this has me thrown for a loop. I feel like the mirror is lying to me, but I know it's not. That is downright depressing.

Side note - I wish I was that person who embraces these new curves. My husband certainly loves them. I envy all of those mid-size and plus-size influencers who are killing it and looking fabulous in the process. I'm not there, yet.

I'm trying. I really am. But I could do more. I know that. I love sugar (and my daughter is a budding pastry chef). Sugar makes me feel better, but worse at the same time. I probably need to start lifting weights. We will get into the science of it all, but it all boils down to hormonal changes and muscle loss. We start to lose muscle at a rapid pace when we are in our forties. When you lose muscle mass, you lose a lot of your ability to burn fat. The first place you gain is the fat around your midsection.

Check. Check. And check.

Side note - This type of fat is called subcutaneous and/or visceral fat. I thought fat was fat?! Subcutaneous fat is the fat that lives just under your skins surface - the jiggly stuff. Visceral fat is firmer and located deep, beneath the abdominal wall. Visceral fat is a dangerous type of fat. Oddly enough, visceral fat is much easier to lose than subcutaneous fat.

Here is the thing... I'm tired (another chapter) and sometimes completely unmotivated. I want to exercise more. I would love to have the ability to play tennis more often, but my joints hurt (again, another chapter).

(Long) Side note - I have a pretty extensive list of past injuries. All sports-related. When I was 18, I had surgery on my wrist from tennis. I stopped playing. I returned at 29, briefly, until I went for a tennis ball and completely severed my ACL. I stopped playing. I told myself that I would never play again. Fast-forward... My daughter gets into soccer, so I start playing more soccer with her. One day, we were playing in the rain, barefoot (something we always did). I planted, to take a shot, slipped, and fell in the shape of a W. Things popped. I knew it wasn't good. I ended up tearing four ligaments, two in each knee along with meniscal tears in both knees. Luckily, three out of the four ligaments (mcl, mcl, lcl, and pcl) healed on their own. I ended up having surgery to repair my torn meniscus, and I still have a partial ACL tear in my right knee. I have been told by 2 orthopedics that my knees will probably prevent me from playing.

But I did it!! I returned to tennis two years ago, in the middle of Peri, knowing I probably shouldn't. I started playing and I loved it. At this point in my life, I'm willing to take the risk. I have also found out that when I play, I'm happier. End of story.

It's a pretty rough cycle, though. I play and then I hurt. These joint pains are real, and they aren't just my knees. They are my elbows and wrists, and sometimes my shoulders. If it were up to me, I would play as much as possible, but my body is telling me differently.

I hope that as I get further into Meno, it will get easier and less painful.

Back to weight gain… Is it inevitable? Maybe? Can you do something about it? Absolutely!

What can be done?

There are all kinds of trendy diets and injections, but I don't believe in those. For me, I need something that I can stick with for the long haul. I know people swear by the new weight loss drugs, and the evidence is there. They do work! I need something that's going to take me from the short term into the long term. I think that magic weight loss is very short-term. Who am I to say? I would love to lose a quick 20 pounds. I know I would feel better, but my biggest fear is that the weight would come back with a vengeance when I inevitably slip up. But that's me… I've got a bit of Sophia Loren in me.

"I'D MUCH RATHER EAT PASTA AND DRINK WINE THAN BE A SIZE 0."

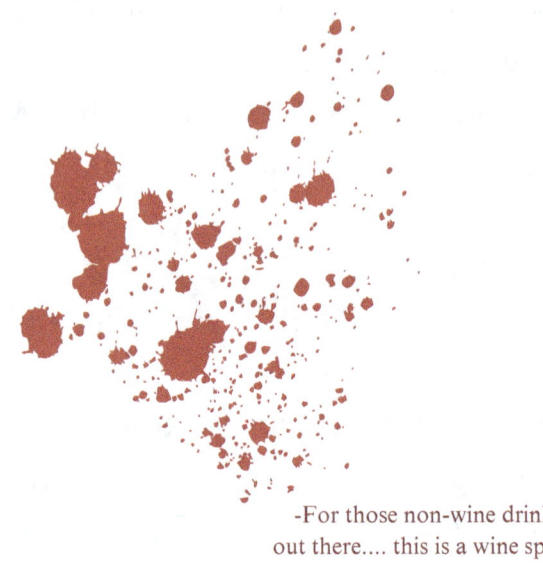

-For those non-wine drinkers
out there.... this is a wine splatter,
or what I like to call "wine art."

Preach, Sophia!!

You know, I'd be happy with a size 10. Shit, I'd be ecstatic with a size 10! At a size 12, I'm not uncomfortable with my body. Peri has definitely made my weight distribution shift. This stomach excess has got to go!!

My husband and I did a dry January. Although he does not drink a lot, I would say that he drinks more than I do. For example, when we open a bottle of wine, I will have a glass maybe a glass and a half. He will usually finish it.

I've done dry(ish) January, three years in a row now. That science experiment has failed and proved that I don't need dry January. Along with dry January, we also tried to eat a little bit healthier, a Mediterranean diet.

The money I saved on wine, I spent on food. That's an expensive diet! I felt a bit trimmer at the end of the 30 days.

My husband lost about 9 pounds and guess what happened to me?

2 pounds.

TWO FUCKING POUNDS!!!

But I felt good. I was a little less bloated and even a friend commented that I looked skinny (thanks Patsy), but I lost only 2 pounds.

I think I've made the long-term decision that I don't EVER need to give up red wine.

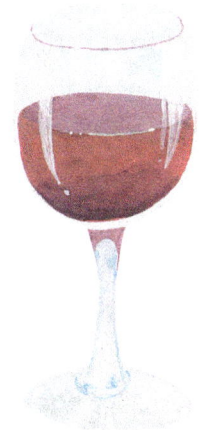

I can't just have wine - I have to pair it with weight training.

There have been extensive studies proving that weight training, especially for pre- and post-menopausal women is essential for weight loss. This makes total sense. During this period of our lives, we lose muscle mass at a rapid pace. The amount of muscle that we have correlates to our ability to lose weight and burn calories. If we have less muscle, we burn less calories.

Hold that thought, while I go work out.

I read an interesting article that I wanted to share.

"Perimenopause and menopause also come with a surprising side effect: dehydration. One study found that changes in estrogen levels can impact women's ability to regulate fluids. It takes more time for their bodies to replenish fluids, putting them at higher risk for dehydration...

Since up to 60% of the human body is water, it's crucial to stay hydrated."

"Water helps regulate body temperature, keeps joints lubricated, and delivers nutrients to cells, among other important functions. It also plays a role in weight gain: The energy provided by water helps the body burn fat.

"One way that water may help with weight is by reducing liquid calorie intake when water is substituted for calorie-containing beverages such as soft drinks, juice, punch, or sweetened teas and coffees," Callahan said.

"Plain water is best, but if you get tired of that, try seltzer or sparkling water without added sweeteners, or add slices of fresh fruit to your water," Callahan said.

https://www.healthywomen.org/your-health/menopause-aging-well/the-secret-to-combating-perimenopause-weight-gain

There are many ways to relieve Peri symptoms, but some are extreme. I'm going to stick with my au naturel way... increase water, weights and decrease sugar.

Most importantly, chat with your doctor. Don't downplay things! They can help or at least give you some options. Perimenopause is a journey, not a destination.

Do what you have to do to be comfortable in your own skin. I'll end this chapter with another quote from Sophia Loren. After all, she is a brilliant woman.

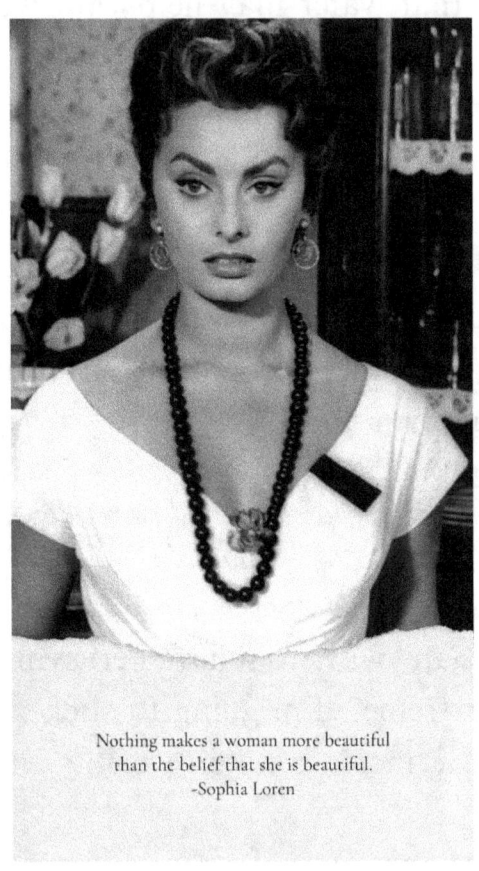

Nothing makes a woman more beautiful
than the belief that she is beautiful.
-Sophia Loren

09

CHAPTER

nine

Chapter Nine
Why does my vagina feel like sandpaper?!

When I began to write this book, the first thing I did was come up with the ideas for the chapters. After I had written a couple of chapters, I shared the pages with the chapter names with my daughter, age 14 at the time.

Let me tell you, she was absolutely mortified when she saw the title of this chapter.

So, Liv… If you have made it this far, skip this chapter. Continue to page 113.

I REPEAT.
SKIP. THIS. CHAPTER!

She was warned.

(I'm even going to jump to the next page).

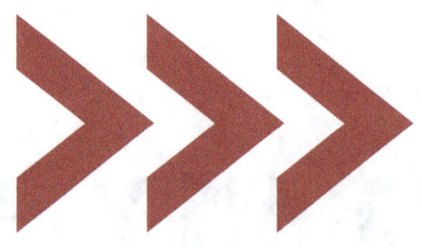

Let's start with what and why? From healthywomen.org, here's some great info:

During menopause, your body changes. Chief among women's complaints: vaginal dryness and other "down there" symptoms. Women agree this condition has a very big negative impact on their lives and self-esteem, using words and phrases like "old" and "less sexual" when describing how it makes them feel.

Why is this happening?

Renowned obstetrician/gynecologist Mary Jane Minkin, MD, a member of the Healthy Women's Health Advisory Council and a champion of getting the word out to women, helps us out by explaining. She says this group of symptoms was previously known as vulvovaginal atrophy or VVA and is now genitourinary syndrome of menopause, also known as GSM or GUSM.

That's a mouthful. What exactly is it?

GSM encompasses a group of bothersome symptoms, like vaginal dryness, itching, urinary urgency, increased frequency, urinary tract infections, and dyspareunia (painful intercourse) that affect more than half of women during and after menopause.

Why does this happen?

Blame hormones. Waning levels of estrogen and progesterone can affect the thin layer of moisture coating the vaginal walls. Suddenly, your vagina is more like a va-DRY-na, one of the most irritating (pun intended) aspects of menopause.

https://www.healthywomen.org/content/article/whats-happening-my-vagina-during-menopause

The article continues to talk about what's normal. Itching, burning, or stinging? All normal?

Of course, Peri would do this to us.

Our once stretchy vajayjay loses its stretch, thanks to the lack of estrogen. Estrogen also keeps bad bacteria in line, so when it decreases, we are more susceptible to urinary issues.

I've been lucky enough to avoid the burning, itching, or stinging, so far. But sex is downright painful. Like the name of the chapter, it feels like my vagina is made out of sandpaper or like 1000 paper cuts.

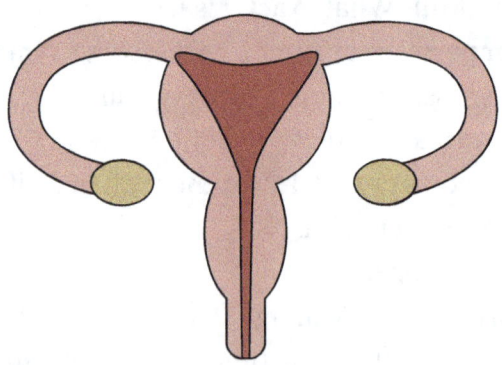

Do you see a uterus or an elephant?
I see a uterus or a martini glass
surrounded by a hug?

I'm going to try to keep this chapter a little modest, because, if this thing ever gets published, I will have family that read it.

The first time it happened, I was shocked and scared. "That's not normal," I thought to myself, but I didn't say anything. Then it happened again and again. Finally, I confided in my husband.

"It hurts, down there, during…"

I couldn't finish the sentence. I was too embarrassed.

"You know, I'm sure we can alleviate that somehow, wink."

My husband… mind is always in the gutter as he tries to make light out of the situation.

Screw it. I am not going to be modest. I promised myself that this book was going to be open, and honest, and candid.

Family - **SKIP** to the next chapter. I grew up Catholic. We don't talk about sex. Ever.

"Don't make fun. This is serious. My vagina hurts, really hurts!" I tell my husband. "I don't know what to do?"

Knowing my keen ability to Google it, he asked if I had researched it.

And he was right. Of course, I researched it. He was going to love the answer.

"There are a bunch of things that help. Time helps. Lube helps. And listen to this... more sex helps."

His response was immediate, typical, and hilarious. He looked up, eyes wide, smiled and said, "Like right now?!"

No, you jackass. I'm trying to be serious and vulnerable! His sentiment did make me smile, but will he ever learn?

• • • • • • • • • • • •

Is there anything else that can be done? Always!

Here's a summary of what's going on.

Of course, hormones are to blame. Specifically, estrogen. Less estrogen lowers blood flow to your vagina. This can cause atrophy... That's when the tissue gets dry and fragile. Your vagina also gets more acidic, which can cause urinary infections.

Remember… Just because this can happen, doesn't mean it will happen.

You can also develop pelvic floor dysfunction. That just means the muscles around your bladder and your vagina spasm. Remember, our lesson on pelvic floor exercises… These again, are important. And here's a scary tidbit: Your pelvic floor might become less stable after Meno, and your bladder and uterus can push on your vagina.

It's normal to avoid things that hurt. I know I do! More sex increases blood flow. More blood flow helps with lubrication and strengthens the tissue.

For so many reasons, I don't feel like sex. It's not just because of the fear of sandpaper. It goes so much deeper than that. *That's what she said.*
All jokes aside, the emotional struggle is real.

For me, I worry about aging, which lowers my self-esteem. The weight gain, of course, doesn't help. The fear of physical pain is constantly on my mind. Will it hurt this time? Not to mention, I feel like my "getting turned on button" is permanently off.

Peri creates a perfect storm to not want sex.

But we have to fight through it! Please know, at least in my husband's case, the weight gain isn't a factor. Quite the contrary, he loves the new curves. I've learned over time that you just have to do it. Sometimes, you have to make yourself because the arousal just isn't there. Once you get started, it gets easier and easier.

Lastly, don't be embarrassed. This is completely normal and affects up to 45% of women going through Peri. (And the other 55% probably stopped having sex altogether)!

Along with more sex, vaginal lubricants and moisturizers (the moisturizers are used for longer-term), low dose vaginal estrogen, and higher dose HT (hormone therapy) can all help or alleviate issues.

What are other ways to help with low libido?
Some women swear by reading smut or erotic novels. "Sexy literature" can help you get out of your head, so you can get into the sheets. Try it. It can't hurt!

Some prescriptions claim to help with a low sex drive. Chat with your doctor about those. Keep in mind that certain medications, specifically SSRI antidepressants can cause a low sex drive.

Talk and sex therapy can certainly help. Sometimes, the simple act of talking about a problem can help solve the issue.

Exercise has been proven to boost libido. It not only increases testosterone levels, but exercise enhances blood flow in the body, stimulating arousal.

Studies have shown that yoga can help with low libido, arousal difficulties, orgasm difficulties, as well as pain during sex.

For me, it's simple. A little bit of yoga, a ton of Kegel exercises, and an attempt at more sex has definitely helped. Also, talking with my husband normalized it.
If the pain doesn't improve, see your doctor.

Peri is trying to take me down, but I won't let her!

P.S. Wine helps.

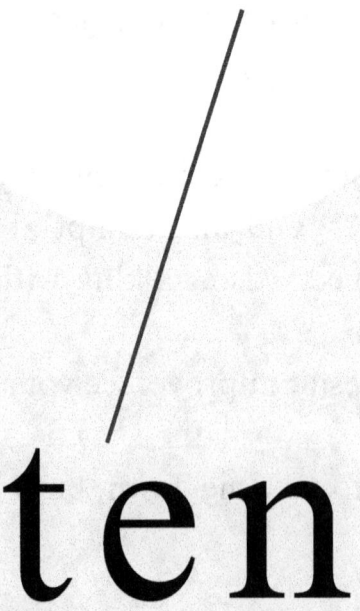

10

CHAPTER

ten

Chapter Ten
Find My Phone

Brain fog, Meno-brain, Cognitive dysfunction, Peri-cloudiness, whatever you want to call it, it is 100% real.

I think brain fog was one of my first symptoms. I didn't realize it at the time. In my early 40s, I found myself searching for words at the end of the sentence. These words weren't readily available, and I had to think about them in order to say them. Normally, we talk. Our brain and our mouth work side-by-side. Normally. It was pretty scary at first. I even asked my doc, who assured me that it is very normal for middle-aged women especially, to have this complaint.

Remembering names has always been difficult for me. Peri has made it more of a challenge. But once I remember your name, I still may forget it. Blame Peri.

Is short-term memory affected more so than long-term memory? We will get to the science of it all, but for me, it seemed that way.

Find My Phone has been a complete godsend. I cannot tell you how many times I lose my phone, sometimes in a day. It's really due to absentmindedness. I will go into my closet, get dressed, and leave my phone there. I will do a load of laundry and leave the phone on a pile of towels. I will pass the couch and put my phone on the arm of it. I will go outside to watch the hummingbirds and leave my phone on the chair. I will go into the store and leave my phone on the car phone dock. I'm sure you are seeing a pattern here?!

Needless to say, I lose my phone a lot. If only my other brain fog issues were easily solved by Find My Phone. I wish.

I lost my wedding ring once. Let's call it misplaced and not lost. I knew that I didn't *actually* lose it. I knew that it didn't fall down the drain, get swept up in the vacuum, or get left somewhere. I knew, in the depths of my brain, that I took it off and put it down somewhere.

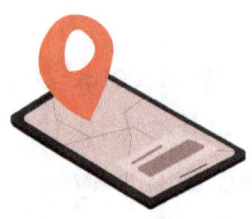

Months went by. I didn't tell my husband because I assumed that I would find it. I even said the old Catholic prayer of St. Anthony,
"Tony, Tony, look around, something's lost and can't be found." If you know, you know.
One day, I was searching in my closet and kept repeating the saying/prayer because why not? It couldn't hurt.

No luck. Another month went by. I started to worry because I knew that my husband and I had a business trip coming up with formal events. You see, normally, I don't wear my diamond every day. I might wear my wedding band, but I save the diamond ring for special occasions.

On Prime Day (Amazon, of course), I even bought a lab-made diamond that closely resembled my ring. Oddly enough, I absolutely love that ring.

When I first realized that I misplaced my ring, I casually brought it up in a conversation with my hubby. It was a 10-second, forgettable conversation. Fast forward to a week before our trip... "Did you ever find your ring?"

Shit. Now I had to tell him.

"No," I said, full of shame. "I know it's not gone. You have to trust me on that. I've searched a lot of the house without much luck, but I know I'm going to stumble upon it."

I went into my jewelry box, and I got the fake.

"What do you think? It's just a replacement until I find the real one."

He shook his head. Not in an angry way. Not even in a disappointed way, just in a Find My Phone kind of way. I was relieved, but I wasn't ready to give up.

Our business trip took us to a tropical location. Naturally, I brought my camera bag.

Side note - Reminder, I am a photographer.

After snapping a few shots of the sunset, I wondered if I packed my adapter (that connects my camera to my phone).

I didn't pack that, but lo and behold, you guessed it... I found my ring!

I couldn't believe it. I wasn't even looking for it. I silently thanked St. Anthony.

It was in the pocket of my camera bag. I must've been taking photos and at some point, my hands got swollen. I took my ring off and stowed it in my bag. Of course, I don't remember that. But it makes complete sense. I can just hear Peri's maniacal laugh. I'm not going to dwell on the fact that Peri is a twat, because I found my ring.

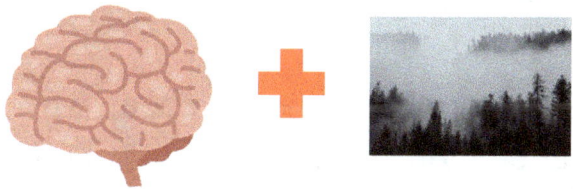

Those are my stories. I wonder what I am forgetting?

Brain fog is one of the most common Peri symptoms. But why? By now, you should know the answer to that question. Estrogen, that's why! Well, not just estrogen, but the lack of estrogen certainly fuels the fire. Studies have shown that menopausal brain fog is due to three main factors: sleep, stress, and hormones.

It seems like a twisted hamster wheel or a nightmare-nonstop revolving door. Your lovely hormones, primarily estrogen, push you. You lose sleep and stress about the chaotic nature of your body. You stress about not sleeping and you sleep less.

I don't know about you, but I need a good 7-8 hours of sleep to feel "rested."

Peri has other plans (see Chapter 13 - Hello 2 am).

The science behind the "why" of brain fog is somewhat inconsistent. One article, from 2021 stated it as such,

"There is a lot of speculation about why some women suffer more from menopause brain than others. It may be related to estrogen levels, or to the interaction between hormone levels and neurotransmitters in the brain in individuals. It is also suggested that lifelong brain health habits (intellectual activity or physical exercise) provide some protection of brain function."

www.theguardian.com/society/2021/oct/10/menopause-brain-the-inability-to-think-clearly-is-not-all-in-your-mind

The Harvard School of Medicine stated that Peri insomnia, specifically waking up because of hot flashes and night sweats, was a leading cause of Meno-brain.

In another interesting study, there is an association between loss of verbal memory skills (being "lost for words") and the severity of hot flashes. One study showed that the women who experienced the most hot flashes in a day also had the worst scores for verbal memory performance. However, even if there are no other Peri symptoms, memory can still be affected by the drop in hormone levels.

https://www.healthcentral.com/article/memory-problems-and-menopause-hot-flashes

Most evidence states that up to two-thirds of Peri women have some sort of cognitive impairment. 66%?!! Why aren't we studying this more?

For me, it's minor and some days are worse than others. Just yesterday, I made my espresso, stirred in my one packet of Splenda, only to take a drink and there was no sugar in it. Brain fog. Later in the day, I did it again! I've adapted, or at least tried to adapt to my new brain. I do notice that if I sleep well, the following day I seem sharper. Maybe that's in my mind?

When the brain fog first started, like many women, I feared the worst... Dementia.

After much research, I learned a very promising tidbit. Brain fog is temporary. What a relief!

Dr. Kling from the Mayo Clinic stated, "We don't have enough studies to say hormone therapy is definitely going to treat those, but many women, once their hot flashes and night sweats are better controlled, their sleep is better, their mood is better. Because they're on treatment for their menopause, they'll notice improvement in their cognitive complaints too," she says.

The good news, brain fog appears to be temporary. Dr. Kling says tests for brain fog after the menopause transition do show improvement. Check with your clinician to find out what treatment is right for you.

https://newsnetwork.mayoclinic.org/discussion/mayo-clinic-minute-does-menopause-cause-brain-fog/

If you are concerned about your cognitive symptoms, chat with a doctor. Is there anything that can be done besides hormone therapy? There have to be women out there, like me. My symptoms are mild to moderate, and as much as they are an annoyance, they haven't decreased my quality of life. I'm good. I'm annoyed, tired, and sweaty, but I don't know that I am ready for hormone therapy.

At home, what can be done?

Do puzzles. Find a type of puzzle you enjoy - Jigsaw, word puzzles like Scrabble or Words with Friends or crossword, number puzzles like Sudoku or KenKen, play board games like chess. Try a new creative hobby such as painting, photography, creative writing, or learning to play a new instrument.

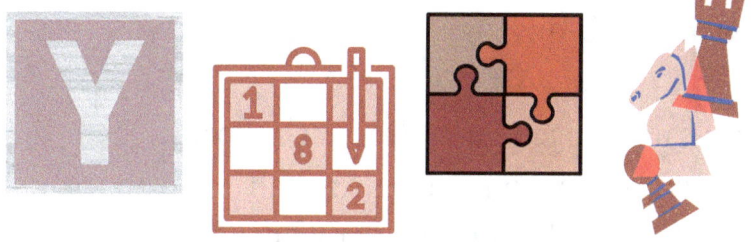

Try to learn a new language. Duolingo and Babbel are free. Parlez-vous francais?

Go for a stroll - sometimes it's as easy as that to lift the fog.

Break large projects down into smaller projects.

Sip orange juice - This is new to me! Compounds called flavonoids in oranges and their juice have a powerful ability to blast brain fog by boosting blood flow to the brain.

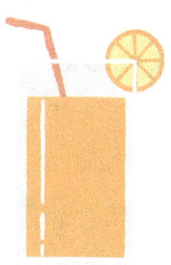

Make a list - as we lose focus because our brains are attempting to juggle 5, 7, or 10 things at once, our brain fog increases.

Change your environment, especially if you work from home. Sometimes carrying your computer to a different room in your house or standing on your front porch to talk on the phone is all it takes to banish Peri brain fog.

Here's a strange one... Grab a cold can.
Just wrapping your hand around a bottle or can that's been chilling in the fridge provides an almost instant brain boost.

Drink more water. Your brain is 75% water, so even the smallest amount of dehydration can cause brain fog.

Eat healthy foods and fats with omega-3s. To support your cognitive health, add more vegetables, fruits, legumes, nuts, beans, grains, cereals, oily fish (salmon, herring, anchovies, mackerel), and unsaturated fats (olive oil, avocado, nuts) to your diet.

Get enough rest - *easier said than done.*

Lack of sleep causes stress and stress causes a lack of sleep. Give yourself time to relax before bed. Try yoga or meditation, even five minutes can prove beneficial. Hot flashes and night sweats are going to happen, but you can create a cooler environment.

Set your thermostat to 68 to 70°. Trust me, you will thank me. Dress lightly, if any clothes at all! Avoid heavy, duvets or blankets.

Steer clear of large meals, caffeine, nicotine, or alcohol directly before bed.

Side note - A glass of red wine with dinner, for me, definitely has relaxing properties.

Supplements - There are a ton of supplements that you can take for cognitive health. There is some evidence to suggest that ginkgo biloba can support short-term memory and help maintain normal brain function. Again, talk to your doctor.

So... That was a lot of information that I just gave you. Thanks for hanging in there!

I'm going to end this chapter with some of the half-brained things that I sometimes do.

I brush my teeth before my shower at night. Sometimes I let the sink water run while I'm in the shower. Apparently, I forgot to turn it off.

Just the other day, I went to play tennis. I came back from my match (two hours later), and my car door was open. Apparently, I forgot to shut it.

I've been known to leave a burner on low after cooking.

You've already read about me losing my phone. This might be an exaggeration, but I feel like this happens every day.

While I have navigation on in my car, I still make a wrong turn.

Side note - Keep in mind, I can still sing every part of Queen's, *Bohemian Rhapsody* or *We Didn't Start the Fire* by Billy Joel.

Every so often, I pour the detergent in the softener spot, and the softener in the detergent spot. That's a bitch to undo.

Every day, I go into a room and say to myself, "What am I doing in here?" Sometimes it comes to me, sometimes it doesn't.

Creatively substituting one word for another, because for the life of me, I can't remember that word in that moment.

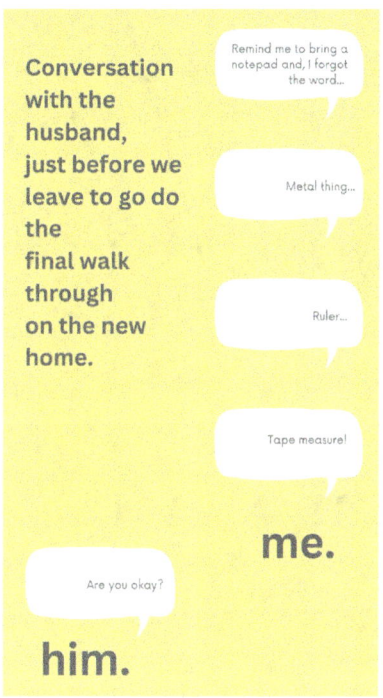

Side note - You might be in Perimenopause if you find yourself searching for words. Somehow, I can't find the word 'tape measure,' but the word 'fuck' rolls right off the tongue.

Just a friendly reminder... THIS IS NORMAL, and this is temporary. Hang in there.

11

CHAPTER

eleven

Chapter Eleven
Head, Shoulders, Knees and Toes (knees and toes)

For me, it's more like neck, elbows, knees, and back.

My aches and pains are definitely one of the more recent symptoms of Peri.

At first, I thought it was just me. It was a logical assumption. I've played a lot of sports and sustained a lot of injuries in my years. My knees started hurting first, mostly during and after tennis.

I wasn't worried. I've got bad knees with torn ligaments. Of course, they are going to hurt. Plus, I'm getting older and have put on a few pounds. Competitively running around after a yellow ball should hurt my knees! After I play, I normally ice them, sometimes take Advil, and I usually take an Epsom salt bath. The pain is short-term. I quickly figured out that I could play tennis, but I couldn't play back-to-back days. I need at least a two-day rest between playing. As long as I do that, my knees are good. Most of the time.

Then my right elbow started to hurt. Again, I was playing tennis, and tennis elbow is very common. I wasn't alarmed or concerned or thinking anything besides, this is what happens when you take 20+ years off of a sport and jump right back in.

The lightbulb finally went off when my left elbow started hurting. Generally, I don't use my left arm for tennis. For those who know the game, I rarely use a two-handed backhand, so my left arm isn't engaged.

At this point, both of my knees hurt, and both of my elbows hurt. I dove in and did some research and quickly found out that joint pain is extremely common during Peri and Meno.
"I feel like I'm falling apart!" I would tell my husband.

The morning after a tennis match, I get out of bed and walk like I'm 90. Everything is so stiff. My muscles are extremely tight and my joints ache, specifically my knees.

Some days are worse than others. Some days I have no pain at all. It's random and it's frustrating.

I started doing extensive research on anti-inflammatory diets. In theory, I could help my inflammation and my pain by limiting inflammatory foods.

Think greens, reds, oranges, and blues.

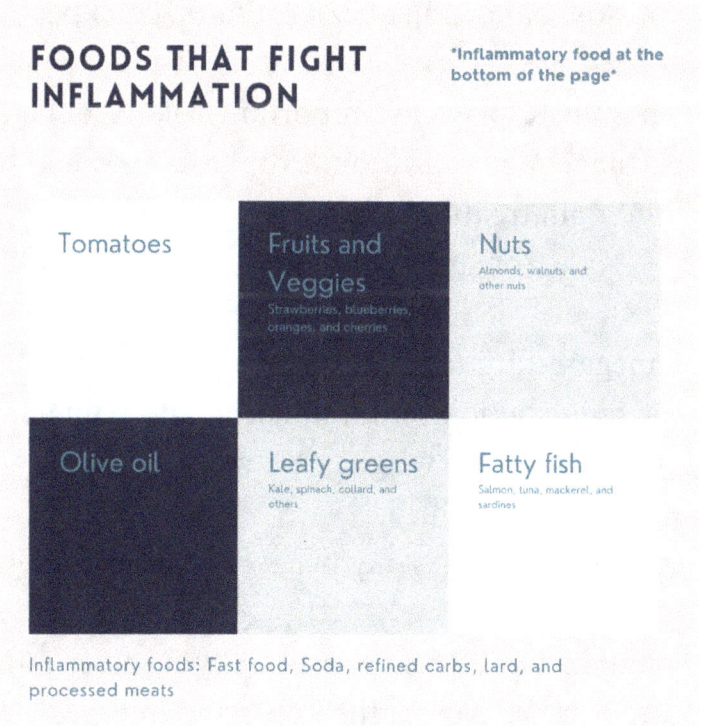

FOODS THAT FIGHT INFLAMMATION

Inflammatory food at the bottom of the page

Tomatoes

Fruits and Veggies
Strawberries, blueberries, oranges, and cherries

Nuts
Almonds, walnuts, and other nuts

Olive oil

Leafy greens
Kale, spinach, collard, and others

Fatty fish
Salmon, tuna, mackerel, and sardines

Inflammatory foods: Fast food, Soda, refined carbs, lard, and processed meats

Fun fact - Coffee, which contains polyphenols and other anti-inflammatory compounds may fight inflammation!

Side note - Red wine for the heart. Coffee for inflammation. I can do that.

- Phytoestrogens are plant-based compounds that act as weak estrogens in the body. They help to balance hormones and alleviate unpleasant symptoms like joint pain.
  - Soy, oats, mung beans, alfalfa, chickpeas

- Vitamin K plays an important role in bone and cartilage mineralization. Proper levels could help joint pain treatment.
  - Kale, tomatoes, pumpkin, parsley, kiwi

- Omega-3 fatty acids have been shown beneficial for reducing joint inflammation and pain as well as improving weight bearing, especially in women with arthritis.
  - Walnuts, flax, oily fish, soybeans, olive oil

- Vitamin D deficiency, especially in older adults, can produce pain in the joints and muscles.
  - Eggs, mushroom, tuna, salmon, carrots
  https://www.palomahealth.com/learn/joint-pain-perimenopause-menopause#:

Preventing excess weight gain is a biggie. I know first-hand that this is easier said than done. It's a struggle, every day.

Peri is an uphill battle with so many hurdles... aches, pains, and weight gain.

At least, it has been for me.

I gain weight... I eat less (and better). Cut out wine and work out more often.

Little to no change. The workout (tennis, pickleball, and walking) makes me ache for days. But I can handle physical pain.

The pain keeps me up at night, as do the hot flashes and general insomnia.

I'm exhausted. I'm stressed because I'm exhausted. My stressed nature (due to insomnia, brain fog, and general achiness) causes my cortisol to rise and make me gain more weight.

Oh, and don't forget that when I exercise, I pee myself! It's fucking great.

Here's the advice of doctors: Nutritious diet. There is a lot of hype about the general health benefits of the Mediterranean diet. Regular exercise. Relieve stress *I'm trying.* Try meditation or yoga or try acupuncture. Be careful, the rate of osteoporosis is higher in aging, Peri and Menopausal women. *Just when I think Peri couldn't possibly get any bitchier, now I have to worry about my bones.*

There are supplements out there, like black cohosh, that contain phytoestrogens. These specific supplements should not be used long-term, but they can get you through the worst parts.

There are also natural hormone-regulating supplements that assist the hormonal glands without supplying the body with outside hormones. These can be taken long-term. Most of these include Magnesium, Vitamin D, Zinc, Vitamin B, and Ashwagandha.

Sometimes, we need more. Sometimes the pain can't be managed by natural methods.

Pain relievers, like acetaminophen or ibuprofen, can relieve acute pain. I hate relying on them.

Your doctor might offer corticosteroid injections to reduce inflammation.

Lastly, hormone replacement therapy (HRT).

It's so difficult to know what's best for you. If you're anything like me, you avoid the doctor. I go to my annual check-ups and screenings, like a good patient. For stuff like aches and pains, I don't ask for help. Maybe I should?

But why is this happening? It's always estrogen (and progesterone). The reduction of estrogen and progesterone can lead to inflammation, fluid retention, and increased sensitivity to pain in the joints.

Basically, the three key hormones play a big role in pain, inflammation, and even arthritis. Estrogen protects joints and reduces inflammation. When estrogen drops, the risks of osteoporosis and osteoarthritis can go up. And as testosterone falls, along with estrogen and progesterone, some women find it harder to maintain muscle.

Getting old sucks, doesn't it? Yoga helps!

12

CHAPTER

twelve

Chapter Twelve
Hello 2 AM

I'm no stranger to insomnia. The fact is, I don't think I've ever been a great sleeper. I've always found it easy to fall asleep, but difficult to stay asleep all night. Just when I thought my sleeping couldn't get any worse, enter Peri.

My insomnia (like most other Peri symptoms) seems to come in waves. Long waves of bad sleep, followed by short durations of decent sleep.

How do I characterize bad sleep?
Waking up more than once and not being able to easily go back to sleep. That's my normal night. I pee a lot more now, so that also affects things.

Good sleep is waking up once, going to the bathroom, and then, immediately back to sleep. I love those nights.

Every so often, the stars align, and I sleep through the night (to 6 or 6:30 am). In the last year, I can count on my hand the number of times that happened.

I've gotten used to it. I also love the occasional nap. I've figured out that if I nap, sometimes I actually sleep better that night! It doesn't make sense, but it is true.

My husband, on the other hand, is a sleeper. I'm jealous of his ability to get to sleep in seconds, (literally seconds) and stay asleep all night. He has a gift.

For my insomnia, I do the basics - no coffee or caffeinated beverages after 3 or 4 pm. I do my best to not eat a big meal late at night. I keep my drinking to a minimum. If I have a glass of wine, it's usually with dinner. I've tried melatonin, without luck. I've tried chamomile tea, without luck. I have had success with Epsom salt baths with lavender.

Do you know what really works? I have an audiobook on Audible. For whatever reason, that thing is like a sedative for me. I usually fall asleep within 5 minutes of turning it on. Here's the problem - I have to go to our guest room and sleep there, in order to listen to it.

It works, but I feel guilty for not sleeping in my bed. I usually only resort to the audiobook when my insomnia is extra bad.

I've tried sleeping with headphones, or earbuds in, but that wasn't comfortable. I've tried listening to it on the lowest volume, but oddly enough, my hubby wakes up. I don't want to disrupt his sleep. I should probably just sleep in the other room. I sleep SO well there. But I don't think I want to. That may sound crazy, but my guilt may be the issue? Maybe I'm just a glutton for punishment? *That could be another book, entirely.* I don't think it's either of those things. I think I'm hopeful that one night my insomnia will just disappear.

Peri, will you ever disappear?
I don't think I am that lucky!

I'm not looking for a pot of gold, but I'm tired of being tired! Sometimes it gets to me, and I snap at my loved ones. Other times it gets to me, and I forget where I put my glasses.

I probably need to do a little more to slow the insomnia. But where do I even begin?

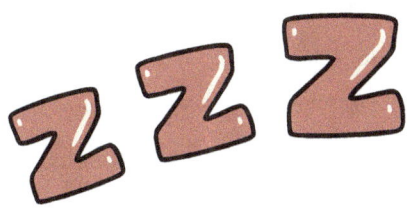

I've read that magnesium can drastically reduce insomnia symptoms. Am I ready to take one more pill? I keep thinking that I'm ready for my own pill pack, but I can't bring myself to buy one. Avoidance - I'm good at that!

But why? Insomnia is a common symptom of Peri and Meno. Of course, I feel like a broken record, but progesterone and estrogen are to blame for some of the lack of sleep.

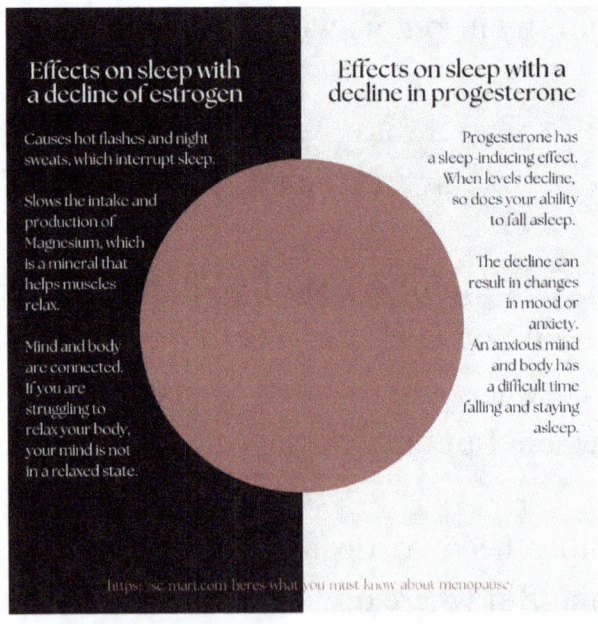

Effects on sleep with a decline of estrogen

Causes hot flashes and night sweats, which interrupt sleep.

Slows the intake and production of Magnesium, which is a mineral that helps muscles relax.

Mind and body are connected. If you are struggling to relax your body, your mind is not in a relaxed state.

Effects on sleep with a decline in progesterone

Progesterone has a sleep-inducing effect. When levels decline, so does your ability to fall asleep.

The decline can result in changes in mood or anxiety. An anxious mind and body has a difficult time falling and staying asleep.

https://sc-mari.com heres-what you must know about menopause

In my case, there are many causes. My hormones, sure, but in this instance, Peri isn't the only bitch to blame. I'm not calling myself a bitch, but I am to blame too. I need to do better. And I will!

Thinking about taking Magnesium? There are so many options - let's break them down.

Magnesium Glycinate - good for those with a deficiency or for those with migraines. Glycine helps with sleep, anxiety, and inflammation.

Topical Magnesium: Magnesium Chloride and Sulfate - Chloride appears to have more healing properties than sulfate. Epsom salt is Magnesium Sulfate.

Magnesium Citrate - Think laxative. This form has the best bioavailability.

Side note - I had to look up the definition of bioavailable. Bioavailability is how well the nutrient is absorbed.

Magnesium Oxide - Inexpensive. Not very bioavailable, compared to other forms. Commonly used for constipation and heartburn.

Magnesium L-Threonate - Best for cognitive brain function or brain fog. No laxative properties. Potentially energizing and best to take in the morning.

Magnesium Malate - Good for fibromyalgia and chronic fatigue. Good bioavailability. Energizing properties make it best to take in the morning.

Magnesium Taurate - Great for migraines and heart-related issues. Shown to reduce heart attacks and promote stable blood sugar.

Side note - Just remember the fewer the ingredients, the better.

What do I mean, I need to do better?

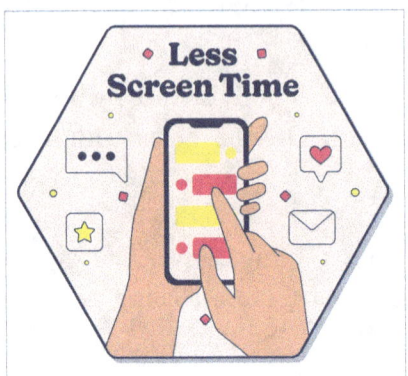

I'm guilty of being on my phone too much. Candy Crush, Wordle, Words with Friends, New York Times games, Amazon... These are all nighttime favorites. Sometimes, I actually think that Candy Crush lulls me to sleep. I realize that sounds absurd, and I realize that I'm probably in total denial. In the words of the brilliant Taylor Swift, "It's me. Hi. I'm the problem, it's me."

Do you know what I'm also guilty of? I'm guilty of having a little 2 AM snack. Again, I swear it helps. It doesn't help my waist, but it helps me get back to sleep. I do my best to have something healthy, or with tryptophan in it.

What exactly is tryptophan? Tryptophan is an essential amino acid used in protein synthesis. Your body cannot synthesize this biomolecular, so you need to get it through diet. This amino acid is used to perform many bodily functions. It helps control mood, sleep, and hunger cycles. Read that again!!

IT HELPS CONTROL MOOD, SLEEP, AND HUNGER CYCLES

It is a building block for many neurotransmitters and hormones.

Let's get back to that mood, sleep, and hunger cycles part. Our bodies use tryptophan to produce important molecules, such as melatonin and serotonin.

The concentration of tryptophan in your brain controls the rate of serotonin synthesis.

LOW TRYPTOPHAN = LESSER RATE OF SEROTONIN SYNTHESIS

Low serotonin may lead to insomnia, depression, and/or anxiety.

And here I was thinking tryptophan was just a Thanksgiving dose of drowsiness.

Because the list is just too long, here are some food categories, and food highest in tryptophan.

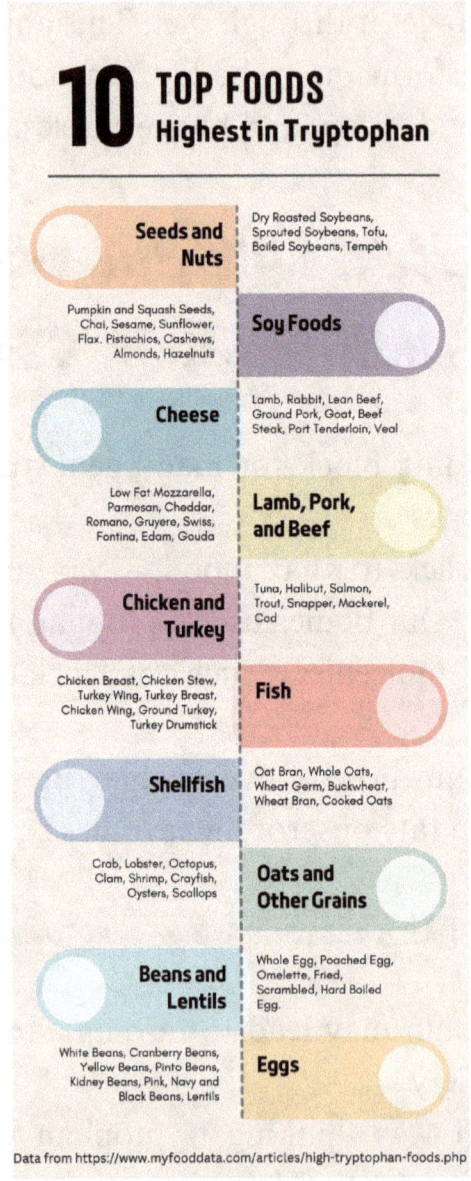

10 TOP FOODS Highest in Tryptophan

Seeds and Nuts
Dry Roasted Soybeans, Sprouted Soybeans, Tofu, Boiled Soybeans, Tempeh

Soy Foods
Pumpkin and Squash Seeds, Chai, Sesame, Sunflower, Flax. Pistachios, Cashews, Almonds, Hazelnuts

Cheese
Lamb, Rabbit, Lean Beef, Ground Pork, Goat, Beef Steak, Port Tenderloin, Veal

Lamb, Pork, and Beef
Low Fat Mozzarella, Parmesan, Cheddar, Romano, Gruyere, Swiss, Fontina, Edam, Gouda

Chicken and Turkey
Tuna, Halibut, Salmon, Trout, Snapper, Mackerel, Cod

Fish
Chicken Breast, Chicken Stew, Turkey Wing, Turkey Breast, Chicken Wing, Ground Turkey, Turkey Drumstick

Shellfish
Oat Bran, Whole Oats, Wheat Germ, Buckwheat, Wheat Bran, Cooked Oats

Oats and Other Grains
Crab, Lobster, Octopus, Clam, Shrimp, Crayfish, Oysters, Scallops

Beans and Lentils
Whole Egg, Poached Egg, Omelette, Fried, Scrambled, Hard Boiled Egg.

Eggs
White Beans, Cranberry Beans, Yellow Beans, Pinto Beans, Kidney Beans, Pink, Navy and Black Beans, Lentils

Data from https://www.myfooddata.com/articles/high-tryptophan-foods.php

My personal favorites on this list are - pumpkin seeds (I roast and toss a big batch with salt, pepper, and garlic powder), almonds, string cheese, soybeans, oatmeal, hard-boiled egg, and a few things in the fruit category that aren't on the list - banana, orange, and dried apricots.

A snack, accompanied by some light stretching, really seems to help me get back to sleep.
When I can't sleep, sometimes I laugh and think of the first two lines from, *The Sound of Silence,*
"Hello darkness, my old friend. I've come to talk with you again."

Side note - If you don't get that reference, I envy your youth and your estrogen!

Part of me wishes that I could be a little more productive when I can't sleep. Truth be told, I feel like it would wake me up more, if I started laundry, edited photographs, or if I wrote in this book. I usually try so hard to get back to sleep. The last thing I am thinking about is chores.

Insomnia sucks. It gets to you. The physical exhaustion leads to mental exhaustion. The mental exhaustion leads to cracks in the psyche.

Eventually, those cracks break. I usually give my husband a warning when I start to feel the exhaustion creeping in.

"It's been a bad few weeks of sleep, and I'm just so tired. So, if I snap at you, I really am sorry."

And I am.

I know it's coming. As much as I try to prevent it, sometimes I can't.

You've heard me say it before. Peri is a bitch. Sometimes, Peri turns me into a cranky bitch.

Last night, I had a relatively good night. I went to bed at a normal time, for me, which was 11 o'clock. I immediately fell asleep. I woke up at 1:53 AM, *not surprised at all by the time.* Tossed and turned for a few minutes. After realizing that I wasn't going to be able to sleep, I got up. I played tennis that night and my hamstrings were extremely tight, so the first thing I did was stretch. I opened up the fridge and looked for some sort of inspiration. I wasn't really hungry, but it's almost like a placebo effect. That little snack helps me return to sleep.

Side note - I don't know it is about that particular time, but I wake up within 10 minutes of 2 am, most nights.

String cheese it is.

I washed the string cheese down with water, took a minute to use the restroom, and then back to bed. It took me a couple of minutes, but I fell back to sleep. I woke up again around 5:30 AM. At this point, my faithful Black Labrador, Indy, knew that it was breakfast time. She normally eats around 6:30 AM, but she also knows that if I wake up after 5 AM, she's getting an early meal. I fed her, took her out, and 10 minutes later I was back to sleep. I woke up 90 minutes later and I was up for the day.

That was a good night for me.

I wish most nights were like that. Like I said before, insomnia comes in waves, ebbs, and flows. Right now, the waves are rough, but I know the tides with change soon.

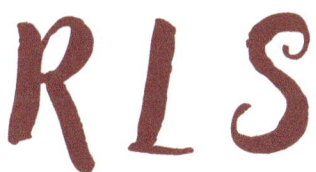

If you know what that stands for, chances are you suffer from it: Restless legs syndrome.

I have it. My mom has it. My aunt, my mom's sister has it. As of late, my daughter has it.

Many studies show there is a link between RLS and Peri/Meno. Mine has nothing to do with Peri, although I think Peri has made it worsen.

The relationship between Meno and RLS is interesting. First off... What is Restless legs syndrome, and what causes it? RLS is a brain, nerve, and sleep condition that causes a strong, nearly irresistible urge to move your legs. It's a condition in which one has feelings of "pulling, searing, tingling" beneath the skin, and the muscles, usually in the calf area (Mine is in the hamstrings).

Restless legs syndrome can run in families. It usually occurs under 40 years of age, if it's gene related. Low levels of iron in the blood may lead to a fallen dopamine, triggering RLS and those achy legs at night. If you are in Peri and you are experiencing heavy periods, you may want to get your iron levels tested by your GP.

Magnesium is also for nerve and muscle function. Deficiency may cause nerve problems.

https://my.clevelandclinic.org/health/diseases/9497-restless-legs-syndrome

Is Restless legs syndrome caused by Meno and Peri? There are different schools of thought here. Interestingly, a 2007 study published in the US Menopause Societies Journal reported that 53% of women over the age of 44, who suffered sleep problems (possibly linked to Peri), also suffered with RLS. As our female hormones, estrogen and progesterone fluctuate, leading up to Meno, it is thought that loss of estrogen impacts the muscle's ability to relax.

www.positivepause.co.uk/menopause-blog/restless-legs-menopause-ruining-menopause-sleep

Sidenote – This adds up. On the nights that I play tennis or pickleball, my hamstrings are usually jammed up. They are tight and tired. Those nights are definitely worse for my RLS.

Everything seems to be linked, somehow.

By now, you've probably realized that I take the natural approach to solving my Peri and Meno problems. Specifically, for RLS, I take both magnesium and iron nightly. My blood work, with the added supplements, comes up with normal levels iron. Bloodwork annually is a must!

There are certain things that you can take that help RLS. Medicines that increase dopamine in the brain have proven, in many cases to treat or lessen RLS. Short-term side effects of these medications are usually mild and include nausea, lightheadedness, and fatigue. However, they also can cause issues with impulse control, such as compulsive gambling and other addictions. They can also cause daytime sleepiness. I think, for those reasons alone, I've chosen not to go that route.

Medicines affecting calcium channels, like Gabapentin, work for some people. Muscle relaxants and sleep medicines help you sleep better at night, but they don't completely eliminate the leg sensations.

I've made a choice to deal with it. In my mind, it's a minor enough symptom. Though some nights, it doesn't seem very minor. At this point, I don't want to change the chemistry in my brain with medication. But that's me! I've also made a choice to play racket sports at night, knowing that it will worsen my RLS. I would rather keep active and deal with the consequences.

There are a lot of successful home remedies. Warm or cold compresses can be soothing. Heated or cold pads can be effective because they create a new sensation for the brain to process. This reduces the sensation produced by RLS.

If compresses aren't your thing, a hot bath or shower can relieve symptoms. Hot water opens up your blood vessels and aids circulation. I usually toss some Epsom salt in my late-night bath to give me a boost of magnesium. Getting more iron in your diet helps on many levels. Certain things trigger RLS, so these are to be avoided, especially before bedtime: Nicotine, alcohol, sugar, and caffeine.

Side note- I can do three out of four. But damnit, Peri! Please don't make me give up my red wine.

Exercise within reason. Too much exercise can trigger RLS, but a mild to moderate walk in the evening can do a lot to relieve your symptoms.

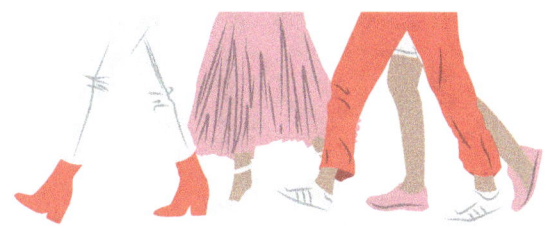

155

Remember, it's OK to seek help. Sometimes, RLS can be debilitating. Lack of sleep can cause depression and anxiety. If that's you, see your doctor. Find one that listens. I've found that my gynecologist is a great source of support and medication (both herbal and prescription). Sleep is so crucial.

After talking with my doctor and weighing the pros and cons, I've learned to adapt to my insomnia. I also live with a very flexible lifestyle. As a photographer, I make my own hours. Writing this book is done when inspiration strikes, or free time is plentiful. I have the luxury of always being able to take a nap, if needed. I'm thankful for that. It's one of the deciding factors behind my decision to not take medicine for insomnia.

So, cheers ladies (and men who are reading) to a good night's rest.

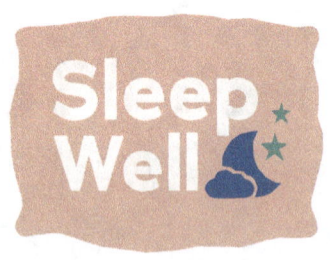

13

C H A P T E R

thirteen

Chapter Thirteen
Is my phone font abnormally large?

Yes. In answer to that question, yes, my phone font is abnormally large. My text font is laughable. It's the largest font setting. It didn't used to be that way. In the last year or two, my eyesight has noticeably changed.

Did you notice that this book is presented in a fairly large font? That is by design. It's so you can read it. It's also so I can read it. I hate readers (the glasses). I'm in denial. I keep telling myself I don't need them. Wrong. I absolutely need them!

This is going to be a relatively short chapter because it's quite simple. Peri and particularly Meno can affect vision. Ready for a cold, hard truth? Chances are, it might not be Meno. It might just be your age. It's official. I'm old.

Can you read the bottom row?

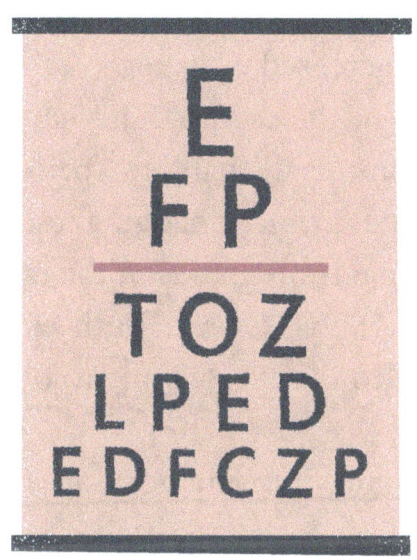

Go to any restaurant, especially one that is dimly lit, and take a look around. I've joined the "Reader's Club" because when I have my contacts in or my glasses on, I cannot read small print. It's really a middle-aged club that I was not ready to join. I thought I had more time.

Not so much.

My actual eye prescription hasn't changed, but my ability to sharply see fine print has VERY much changed.

Let's go to the why of the question. During late Peri, the considerable drop in estrogen levels can lead to increased water retention and inflammation of the cornea. This can affect vision and make it more difficult to focus on close-up objects or fine print. Changing estrogen levels, negatively impacts oil glands in the eyes, as well as the elasticity of the cornea. Both can affect how light travels into the eye, leading to blurry vision.

Here we go again. Fucking hormones.

That's not all! Those symptoms can be accompanied by extra tearing, dry eyes, and light sensitivity. Wait! There's more?!

Your eyes can change shape. It sounds crazy, but the change is very slight. Those of you who wear contact lenses might suddenly realize that your contacts don't fit like they used to.

Dry eyes are one of the biggest complaints during Peri. Your eyes are made up of tissues called mucus membranes. These membranes are seriously affected by falling estrogen levels.

Sometimes, on the opposite end of the spectrum, you can also end up with watery eyes. During Peri, we know by now that your estrogen levels are going to fluctuate. Just like the flow of your period, it can also impact the flow of your tears.

Side note: Where is the irony here? Watery eyes? I cry at everything. Now you're telling me that I can have watery eyes for no reason??!! That's messed up.

Another potential effect of Peri/Meno changes is a higher risk of glaucoma. Glaucoma is a disease that damages the eye's optic nerve, usually caused by high eye pressure.

Can we do anything about this?
Be proactive. Get your eyes tested regularly.
Keep your blood pressure in normal ranges. High blood pressure can damage the tiny blood vessels that supply blood to the eyes. This can lead to optic nerve damage.
Balance your hormones, if you can.
Eye drops work wonders.
Make sure you get enough omega 3s, like oily fish. If you're vegetarian/vegan, consider things like flaxseed oil and walnuts.

The next one is news to me...

Eat brightly colored foods. Brightly colored foods contain compounds such as lutein, along with vitamin A. Some examples are carrots, beets, bell peppers, and tomatoes. I remember when I was young, my mom taught me that carrots are good for your eyes. That checks out! Zinc is also really important for eye health.

Last but not least, water. Remember that during Peri and Meno, women get extra dehydrated. Dehydration will affect your eyes, contributing to dry eye and affecting eye pressure.

Okay... Drink water, eat carrots, and go to the eye doctor yearly. Got it.

Side note - Books commonly use 10 to 12-point font. **Not this book.** 14pt font - so readers are optional.

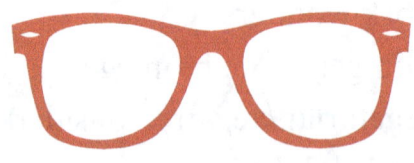

14

CHAPTER

fourteen

Chapter Fourteen
Why am I crying at everything?

Let me preface this chapter by saying that I've always felt like the tiniest bit of an empath. I feel all the emotions around me, and they sometimes affect me.

Side note - I know this is random, but is it affect or effect? Considering my background in college (English), I should know this. It's one of those grammatical instances that I question. Here's the easy answer... Affect is usually used as a verb. Effect is usually used as a noun. You would think that I would remember that! Every time I write the word, I wonder if it's correct?

Once I got into my 40s, I noticed that I was reactively crying often. Now, when I say reactively crying, I mean the tears were my immediate reaction to something. Sometimes, that something is nothing. Sometimes, it's the song. Sometimes, it's a commercial. Sometimes, it's seeing my daughter thrive or seeing my daughter struggle. Sometimes, it's talking about an emotional subject. Sometimes, it's looking at my overly loyal, Black Labrador. She loves so unconditionally, and it makes my eyes water. Let's just say, I get choked up easily.

I've noticed that recently, thinking about sad things doesn't make me cry. Talking about sad things makes me cry.

And when I say cry, I mean tear up. I'm not over here wailing in the corner.

Movies really make me cry. Happy or sad, it doesn't matter. I get all of the feels. I've become a bit of a laughingstock in my family. I'm OK with it. My daughter and husband know that if we turn on a movie, chances are I will tear up. Every time I do, they laugh and shake their heads.

"Mom's crying, *again*," they snicker.

I learned to be prepared. I have sunglasses and Kleenex in my purse, at all times. I'm the person with an inner monologue repeating,

"Don't cry, don't cry, don't cry."

Sometimes, it actually helps.

About eight years ago, I was 100% not prepared. We were on a plane, going somewhere, and I decided to watch, "The Good Dinosaur."

Now, one would assume that this is not a tearjerker. One would assume wrong.

Spoiler alert... When the little boy leaves his dinosaur bestie, and then he howls (like he is calling him back because he's family)... Waterworks. This was not just tearing up. These were giant, rapidly falling tears. You know the kind. Uncontrollable runny nose, you know the one. My husband looked at me as if to say, "What is wrong with you???" I rummaged around in my seat and managed to find the tiny napkin that they gave me on the plane. From that moment on, I was a little better prepared.

For me, being a mom plays into a lot of my tears. I've always felt like there is a physical connection between me and my daughter. I feel her triumphs, and I feel her failures. I feel her anxieties. Sometimes, I feel her annoyance. Of course, I don't feel them like she feels them.

I can remember when she was graduating from Pre-K. She was an early reader and was chosen at their graduation ceremony to read in front of the parents.

She was four and scared shitless. Her face was green, as she walked on stage. I couldn't do anything about it.

One of her amazing teachers picked up on her stage fright and swooped in to ease her anxieties. I watched her from the side stage. It was as if I could read her mind. I could certainly read her emotions.

She was nauseous.
She was anxious.
She felt like she was going to throw up.
And so did I.

She didn't. She rocked it. When she did, I felt her utter relief. In that relief, the tears started flowing.

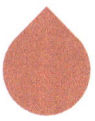

As much as I could write an entire chapter on tears, this chapter goes much deeper than that. Peri is notorious for her wildly changing moods.

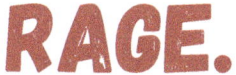

I can remember feeling rage. Blind rage. As much as I can remember the feeling, I don't remember what it was about. It was like a switch was flipped. My husband was the *somewhat* innocent target. I'm sure he did something, that on any other day would slightly annoy me, but not enough to react. But not on that day. Not at that time. I saw red. I hypothetically dreamt of murder. I was so angry at something so small. Of course, at the time, it was not small at all.

I see glimpses of that anger in my daughter.
"What is wrong with you?!"
I asked, thinking that I was not to get an answer from her. Except the one day. I remember it well. In her rage, she also had a moment of clarity. She surprisingly answered the question by saying,
"I don't know."

Sometimes, I feel like my teenage daughter and I are on the same roller coaster. I grew up in Cincinnati, Ohio. Although I'm not one for roller coasters, there is one coaster at Kings Island called, The Racer.

It is a roller coaster with two different directions. You choose whether you want to be on the part of the roller coaster that goes forward, or the part of the roller coaster that goes backward. I always chose backward. I felt less sick that way. That's kind of how I can describe our mother-daughter emotional bond right now. She's getting on and I'm getting off, but our erratic emotions are so similar.

Or should I say, they were so similar. Here is some fantastic news... Once you move through Peri, moods tend to stabilize. It usually means your hormones have plateaued, or you've just accepted your estrogen-free fate.

Someone once accurately described Peri as PMS on steroids.

I really think I could be past all the moodiness. I still get cranky and annoyed. Don't we all? It has less to do with my hormones and more to do with my sunny disposition.

My family swears that my moods have stabilized.

One night, at the dinner table, we were chatting about my moods. "When do you think that happened?"

"Maybe within the last year or so?" Said the hubby.

I was a bit taken aback by that answer. I really thought it was longer.

"Really!? So... It was before or after we moved to Georgia?"

My daughter quickly interjected,

"After. Definitely after." She continued saying, "You were bad, for a minute."

I nearly choked at her response and quickly got (jokingly) offended.

"Me?? You have little room to talk, my moody child."

She shrugged her shoulders and smiled, as if to agree with me. They were probably right. As the bleeding was leaving my body, so was the female rage.

Side note - Everyone talks about a mother's love. No one talks about a mother's rage.

It's not just rage. For some, there's an entire gauntlet of emotions, ranging from anxiety to depression. I have been lucky enough to avoid depression. I have my fair share of anxieties, but they weren't necessarily worsened by Peri.

In doing my research for this little project, changing moods and weight gain are the most common and most complained about symptoms of Perimenopause.

Let's get a little bit more serious here. There's a definite link between Peri and depression. When women go through sudden and intense hormonal changes, like the ones that come along with puberty, postpartum, and Peri, they are at a higher risk for depression, according to mental health experts. The same hormones that control your period, also impact your serotonin. Serotonin is a brain chemical that assists in feelings of well-being and happiness. A big dose of serotonin is like a shot of joyous sunshine. When hormone levels drop, serotonin levels fall. This contributes to increased irritability, anxiety, and sadness.

Studies have shown that women who have been diagnosed with depression in the past are more likely to have depression during Peri.

Falling estrogen and progesterone levels can trigger mood swings, making it more difficult to cope with the stresses and changing emotions.

It's definitely important to chat with your doctor, especially if you have had past episodes of depression, especially postpartum. If you know these emotions are coming, or that there is even a possibility that they might come, you'll be in a better spot to recognize, handle, and treat them. Knowing is half the battle, right? Plus, mood fluctuations are so treatable.

Side note - you should know that I'm writing this chapter between 3 and 4 a.m. I've gotten used to my insomnia. If I can't turn the brain off, I might as well use it.

It's not just the hormones causing the mood swings. They are probably the biggest culprit, but not the only one. It's really everything that comes along with Peri. The insomnia. The weight gain. The hot flashes. These three symptoms alone can cause anxiety, depression, or just a shitty outlook on life.

Everyone has their own story and their own hurdles. Midlife is a time of change, both physical and emotional. Sometimes, there's career pressure, marital stress, aging parents, health problems, and even kids growing up and leaving home (just to name a few). Those pressures bear a big weight and can intensify mood swings and even the possibility of intrusive thoughts and depression.

You know what? It's OK not to be OK. It's normal not to be OK. There's no need to hide in the shadows, alone. You are not alone. This is all temporary and there are things that can be done to help. Please don't be afraid to ask for help!

At the peak of Peri, although I wasn't depressed, I was certainly ashamed. I felt old and ugly and fat. I felt like my brain didn't work and my yo-yo emotions were exhausting.

I knew I had to do something. But what? I knew that if I joined the gym, I would do what I always do... go for a few weeks and then stop. I don't have the best track record when it comes to traditionally working out. What can I say? I'm not a gym person.

Fate stepped in and after many years away, I stepped back onto the tennis court.

It has made so much difference. The tennis court lead me to the pickleball court. I certainly have not lost the Peri weight, but it's leveled out. My joints ache, but I'm happy. I got lucky. I took a small step outside of my comfort zone. I'm better because of it.

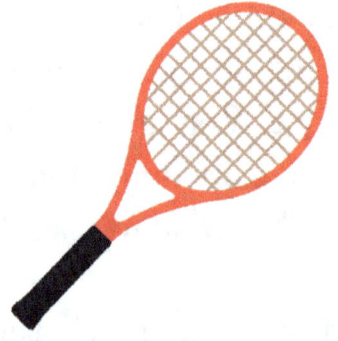

What if you find yourself there? How do you find relief? An educational article on healthline.com listed the following ways:

Accept your anger. Don't bury it. You may want to suppress your anger, so it doesn't inconvenience anyone else. Research shows that "self-silencing" puts you at a greater risk for depression.

Listen to your body and accept that what you're going through is fleeting and may be a result of your body's new hormonal adjustments.

Learn your triggers. These are some lifestyle habits, like drinking too much caffeine or smoking cigarettes, that may trigger anxiety. Dehydration can also make you more prone to mood swings. If your sleep is interrupted by hot flashes, it may be difficult to handle certain emotions.

Take a step back. When you're in the middle of a heated moment, practice taking a step back. Breathe and think about where your emotions are coming from. Don't discourage yourself for being angry, but at the same time, evaluate your anger. Ask yourself, would I be so angry if I were feeling better?
This is all easier said than done.

Meditate. Mind-body therapies, such as meditation and yoga, have been found to have huge benefits for women in Peri. Mindfulness apps are an easy way to spend a couple of minutes a day, at home, meditating. *One free one that I like to use is called Insight Timer.*

Find an outlet. Physical outlets like aerobic exercise, working out, and lifting weights, can help keep you from gaining weight, as your metabolism slows down. Exercise also taps into the serotonin supply that you need to boost and manage your mood. Other outlets, such as gardening, painting, and writing, can help you focus on cultivating a quiet space in your mind.

Take medication, as needed. Talk with your doctor. Low-dose birth control can be prescribed to help even out your moods. Antidepressants can also be taken as a temporary measure to help you feel more balanced. It's not something that has to be permanent, just something to get you through the rough times.

Consider therapy. Sometimes, the simple act of talking about your feelings can help you manage your anger.

https://www.healthline.com/health/menopause/
perimenopause-rage#tips-for-management

Take care of you. Sometimes as women, wives, mothers, employees, or boss babes, we spend a lot of time worrying and taking care of everyone else, but ourselves. I will repeat that. Take care of you.

15

CHAPTER

fifteen

Chapter Fifteen
Hormone Replacement?

HRT (Hormone Replacement Therapy)
If you're anything like me, the idea of hormone therapy scares you. I've read so much about the science of it. It doesn't put me at ease. It actually just brings up more questions.

I haven't been on a birth control pill since my 20s, so my body is not used to any additional hormones. I also feel like it's a band-aid. It may solve your problems temporarily, but eventually, you have to get off of it. You can't be on it forever.

When you get off of it, 2 years down the road, 5 years down the road, 10 years down the road?
What's that like?
Do you go through estrogen withdrawal?

After reading tons of articles, talking to my doctor and to friends who have experienced it, I've opted not to do any sort of hormone therapy. *For now.*
Would I like these symptoms to go away?

Hell, yes!

I'm so sick of not sleeping. I'm sick of gaining weight around the midsection. I'm sick of my sagging skin. My husband is sick of my lack of libido. But HRT does not come without some risk. I can handle the symptoms. As much as I don't like them, and I wish I felt a little better, they are merely a nuisance that I've grown accustomed to.

That being said, I'm still on the fence. It's hard to know what's right, and if the benefits outweigh the risks.

There are definite pros and cons to taking HRT. Before we get into those, what exactly is HRT? Hormone replacement therapy is a therapy with estrogen, progesterone, and sometimes testosterone, which replaces the hormones that your body is no longer making during Peri/Meno.

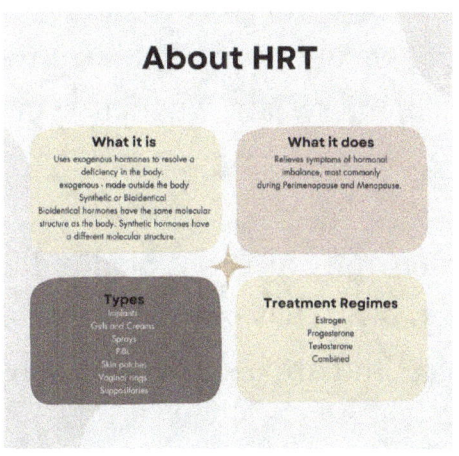

When you talk about HRT, there are a couple of different types. Also, there are different ways the hormones enter your body.

ET is estrogen-only therapy. The lack of estrogen causes the majority of Peri symptoms. ET is often prescribed for women without a uterus, due to a hysterectomy.

EPT is estrogen combined with progesterone. Progesterone is often added to ET to protect women with a uterus, specifically from uterine cancer.

There are generally two ways to take hormone therapy. Systemic products circulate in the bloodstream to all parts of the body. They are available in a pill, patch, gel, emulsion spray (a skin spray that gets absorbed and goes into the bloodstream), or injection. These can be used for hot flashes, night sweats, vaginal symptoms, and osteoporosis.

Local products only affect a localized and specific area of the body. They are available in a cream, ring, or tablet, and are used for vaginal symptoms.

Another form of HRT is testosterone. For women, there is not a single form of testosterone HRT that has been FDA-approved, yet many doctors are still prescribing it. Most women seek testosterone treatment due to low libido and fatigue.

Shockingly, while researching testosterone HRT, information was not easy to find. I'm guessing this is why there is no FDA approval, just yet. TRT (testosterone replacement therapy) is shrouded in mystery, and I find that odd.

Here is what the Cleveland Clinic has to say about low testosterone treatment,

"Treatment for low testosterone can be controversial because low testosterone in women and people AFAB (assigned female at birth) hasn't been well-studied. The U.S. Food and Drug Administration (FDA) hasn't approved any testosterone treatments currently. As there isn't a standard for treatment, providers treat low testosterone in women the same way they'd treat it in men. This can be problematic because women and people AFAB require significantly less testosterone (a much lower dose of medication) than men and people AMAB."

https://my.clevelandclinic.org/health/diseases/24897-low-testosterone-in-women

In summarizing collective research, testosterone therapy is not just for men; it can also be beneficial for women, particularly those experiencing symptoms of hormone imbalance.

Testosterone pellets are a popular method of this type of hormone replacement therapy for women, due to their convenience and effectiveness. However, like any medical treatment, there are potential side effects which include: acne, hair growth on the face and body, hair loss on the head, and weight gain.

Due to a lack of research on long-term safety, testosterone therapy isn't right for women with heart, blood vessel, or liver disease. It's also not for those who've had breast or uterine cancer. If you have a high risk of any of these conditions, talk with a member of your healthcare team about the risks of taking testosterone.

Side note - Outspoken personal opinion here, but testosterone treatment seems questionable and risky. Without doing this research - and it was a pretty deep dive, how can the women going through Peri and Meno be informed? It's frustrating and scary. And the pellets... they are small, rice-sized implants that are inserted subcutaneously, usually in the hip or buttock area. These pellets slowly release testosterone over several months, providing a steady dose of the hormone. I have so many questions... What if they don't work or you have adverse side effects? Do you have to wait it out? From my understanding, that's exactly what you have to do.

Circling back to ET. Let's say you decided on estrogen replacement therapy. The decision-making isn't over. There are many types of estrogen therapy, in many forms – pills, patches, suppositories, and more. The most common form is a pill or a patch,

Estrogen pills are usually taken once a day without food. There are some obvious pros of taking ET in the form of a pill. Pills are easy and convenient. They also lower the risk of osteoporosis. While there are newer ways of getting HRT, oral estrogen is the most studied type of ET.

What are the cons? Estrogen causes a slight increase in the risk of strokes, blood clots, and other problems. When combined with the hormone progestin, the risks of breast cancer and heart attack rise as well. Oral estrogen, like any estrogen therapy, can also cause side effects. These include painful breasts, vaginal discharge, headache, and nausea. Because oral estrogen can be hard on the liver, people with liver damage should not take it. Estrogen is sometimes not well absorbed. It may increase your cholesterol because it is metabolized in the liver.

Another way to get estrogen is through skin patches. Many patches combine estrogen and progesterone. Usually, you wear the patch on your lower stomach, beneath your waistline. You would then change the patch once or twice a week, according to your instructions.

In addition to having the same benefits as the pill form, this type of estrogen treatment has several additional advantages. For one, some find the patch more convenient because you don't have to worry about taking a pill every day.

While estrogen pills can be dangerous for people with liver problems, patches are OK because the estrogen bypasses the liver and goes directly into the bloodstream.

In a 2019 study, The University of Nottingham researchers found that women who use HRT tablets are 58% more likely to develop a blood clot within 90 days than those who did not use HRT. Women who used HRT absorbed through the skin with patches, gels, or creams had no increased risk of blood clots.

https://www.webmd.com/menopause/which-type-of-estrogen-hormone-therapy-is-right-for-you

The disadvantages of the patch are... it's a patch.

The patch itself might irritate the skin where you apply it. Estrogen patches should not be exposed to high heat or direct sunlight. Heat can make some patches release estrogen too quickly, giving you too high of a dose. You can't use tanning beds or saunas while you're wearing an estrogen patch. Also, some users complain that sweat around the patch loosens it.

Other types of estrogen treatment come in the form of creams, gels, and sprays. Most of the gels or creams are applied on the arm.

Because estrogen creams are absorbed through the skin and go directly into the bloodstream, they are safer than oral estrogen for people who have liver or cholesterol problems.

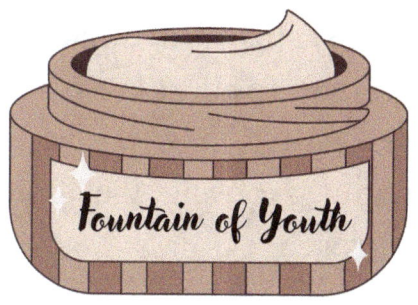

However, estrogen gels, creams, and sprays have not been well studied. They pose the same risk of serious problems, like cancer and stroke. One potential problem with using this type of treatment is that the gel, cream, or spray can rub or wash off before it's fully absorbed. Because the estrogen is absorbed right on the skin, if other people touch these creams or gels, they can get dosed with estrogen themselves.

Side note - Let me get this straight, I can dose my kid or husband with hormones? Interesting...
All kidding aside, I love the idea of a cream because it stays away from the liver. Being able to transfer to someone else is definitely something to keep in mind.

The last type of estrogen treatment is through vaginal suppositories, rings, and creams. These specifically treat women who are troubled by vaginal dryness, itchiness, burning, or pain during intercourse.
Studies have shown that when it comes to treating vaginal symptoms, these treatments are more effective than other forms of estrogen therapy. The advantage is that they can relieve vaginal symptoms without exposing the entire body to high doses of estrogen.

They won't help symptoms like hot flashes. They are for more localized problems. Most doctors do not recommend long-term vaginal estrogen therapy to women who still have their uterus because it may increase the risk of endometrial (uterus) cancer.

https://www.webmd.com/menopause/which-type-of-estrogen-hormone-therapy-is-right-for-you

How do you choose?
When deciding on what type of estrogen therapy to get, work closely with your doctor. The oral form of estrogen is well-studied. Because other forms of taking hormones are newer, there is less long-term evidence.

The full risks of hormone therapy are unclear. If you decide to get HRT, experts collectively recommend that you take the lowest dose, for the shortest time.

I've spoken to many Peri/Meno women about HRT. Most are on the fence and know little about it. Several ladies have said the same thing, "I wish I would have taken it sooner," or "Just do it, you'll feel better." When I hear that, it makes me think twice, but personally, the risks to too high.

Are you confused yet? I know I am!

In doing a deeper dive into hormone therapy, there is traditional hormone therapy, which is what we talked about in the previous pages. Traditional HRT uses synthetic and animal-derived hormones that closely mimic human hormones. Your body then uses them in the same way as your natural hormones.

Enter BHRT or bioidentical hormone replacement therapy. Hormones in BHRT are derived from plant molecules like yams or soy. *So, are they vegan?*

They are called bioidentical hormones, as they are chemically identical to human hormones. Because they are an exact match to the hormones and hormone receptors in your body, your body reacts to them as it would your own natural hormones.

Sounds too good to be true, right? This is where it gets tricky.

"The FDA has approved certain types of bioidentical hormones. Other forms of bioidentical hormones are custom-made by a pharmacist, based on a healthcare provider's prescription. These are compounded, bioidentical hormones."

"The compounded forms have not been tested and approved by the FDA. However, it is often advertised that products that are made from plants are "natural" choices. They are altered in a lab, so they are no longer natural when done with processing. Both the FDA-approved and compounded hormones come in various doses and forms: pills, creams, patches, inserts."

https://my.clevelandclinic.org/health/treatments /15660-bioidentical-hormones

Bioidentical hormones have been controversial, and many are not FDA-approved. That doesn't mean your healthcare provider will rule them out as a treatment option. It's so important to advocate for yourself, have candid conversations with your doctors, and do a little bit of research on your own.

From the extensive research I've done, for my benefit, but also for this little project, I'm still not convinced that HRT is for me. That doesn't mean it's not right for you. My deciding factor? I have a long family history of breast cancer.

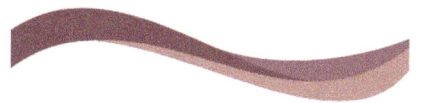

There are many benefits of hormone replacement therapy. For many healthy adults who are experiencing moderate or severe Peri/Meno symptoms, the benefits of using HRT outweigh the potential risks of the treatment.

Medical experts note the benefits of HRT can include relief from moderate to severe hot flashes, relief from vaginal dryness and discomfort, prevention of bone loss and bone fractures, and protection against colorectal cancer. In addition, the American College of Obstetrics and Gynecology notes that otherwise healthy people who are experiencing early Meno or estrogen deficiency may find HRT beneficial.

HRT is recommended on an individual basis. It's not a one-plan-fits-all type of Peri and Meno fix. It's so important to speak to your healthcare provider about the potential benefits and the risks of HRT, based on your symptoms, your medical history, your genetics, and your overall health.

Side note - How can you find a doctor who answers your questions, and takes into account your genetics and medical history? How do you find a unicorn?

Most medical experts agree that HRT is an option worth considering, for healthy adults under 60. It's crucial to point out that years of research have highlighted several potentially serious risks of using HRT. But are those studies outdated?

One of the biggest studies that started in 2002, raised significant concerns, including that some participants had a higher risk of breast cancer, heart disease, stroke, blood clots, urinary incontinence, gallbladder disease, and dementia. Importantly, most of the affected participants were over the age of 60, and over the Meno phase. Since then, scientists and researchers have continued to analyze these findings, as they explore the long-term safety of HRT.

Experts have clarified that the potential risks may be more likely in people who begin HRT at 60 and older, begin HRT more than 10 years after the start of Meno, or have a personal or family history of conditions like cancer and heart disease.

Wow! That was a lot of information. There are so many options to weigh.

I will say it again, talk with your doctor. Find a doctor who really listens. At this point in my Peri journey, my symptoms are a pain in the ass, a nagging nuisance. They aren't ruining my life. But for some women, Peri is debilitating. Whether your symptoms are mild, moderate, or severe, know that you are not alone. There is no shame in talking with your doctor. Let's normalize these conversations.

Side note - Men have it so easy. They just have to deal with a prostate exam and possible erectile dysfunction. Ever wonder why there seems to be more focus on ED than menopause? There are a couple of reasons for this... Historically speaking, research has been male-dominated. Naturally, the researchers are going to focus on something that hits closer to home. Also, there is a huge market for ED treatments, like Viagra and Cialis. When this happens, funding comes pouring in, followed by more extensive research. Hopefully, the current and next generation of researchers are full of brilliant women!

16

CHAPTER

sixteen

Chapter Sixteen
That can't be good?!

I've said that several times to myself, both out loud and in my head.

When I noticed my readers weren't strong enough... That can't be good.
When I bled, so heavily, that two tampons and period undies didn't cover it... That can't be good.
The time when I started counting the number of joints that ached, and it was over 5... That can't be good.
When my occasional insomnia turned into consistent insomnia... That can't be good.
When my heart palpitated, and I felt my first arrhythmia... That can't be good.

The biggest "that can't be good" moment had to be when my periods turned dark red/brown/black. That was more of an "Oh, fuck!" moment - followed by... That can't be good.

Side note - Did you notice that this book is full of text in different shades of red?

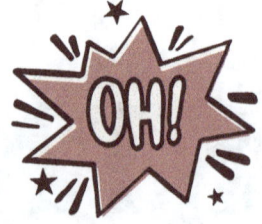

That's what this chapter is about, the first time black blood happened. I was scared to death. I immediately called my doctor. She immediately told me that during Peri, it's normal. If you aren't in Peri, it needs to get checked out.

It was such a visceral memory. I can't remember where my phone is, but I can remember exactly what I was wearing, the season of the year, and my exact feelings at that moment.

As we've talked about before, Meno is technically 12 full, long months without any sort of period. For me, the 12 months before that were crazy.

Estrogen's role is to thicken the uterine lining before ovulation. When estrogen levels become imbalanced, the lining begins to shed irregularly, resulting in light or heavy bleeding, spotting, and missed periods.

When you get into late Perimenopause and skip a period, *and you will,* make sure to talk with your doctor. If you are anything like me, it means you are in the home stretch. How many more times will my uterus shed? Only Peri knows.

If the blood hangs around in your uterus for a while, it turns brown, because of oxidizes. Basically, those dark periods are just old blood.

Should you be concerned about dark brown blood? Call your doctor if it smells bad, if it lasts a long time. or if accompanied by a fever.

During that last year, your flow will probably change colors from the brightest of red to dark reddish/black.

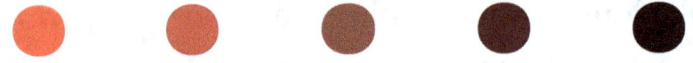

Your cycle will likely be irregular. You may have cramping, but no period. You may have dark, intermittent spotting.

In my last 18 months, the bleeding went from ridiculously heavy to barely there. I would skip a month. I would skip two months. At the very end, I skipped six months, and then I was done.

You're dwindling numbers of estrogen and progesterone causes wild period irregularities.

Freaking hormones! In case you are a numbers person...

Hormones	Stages
Estrogen	Perimenopause Fluctuates unevenly Levels are between 45-854 pmol/L Menopause Levels fall down considerably. Can be as low as 30 pmol/L Postmenopause Levels remain at less than 100 pmol/L
Progesterone	Perimenopause Fluctuates unevenly Normal range is between 5 to 20 ng/mL Menopause Levels rise to a range of 11.2 ng/mL to 90 ng/mL Postmenopause Drops drastically to as low as 1 ng/mL
Testosterone	Perimenopause Fluctuates unevenly Normal range is between 5 to 20 ng/mL Menopause Levels rise to a range of 11.2 ng/mL to 90 ng/mL Postmenopause Drops drastically to as low as 1 ng/mL

https://www.nirvahealth.com/blog/menopause-hormones

Don't fret if your periods turn against you, or if they are so irregular it scares you. It is normal. Of course, just like everything else, talk with your doctor about these changes. It may not be necessary, but it might help you sleep better at night.

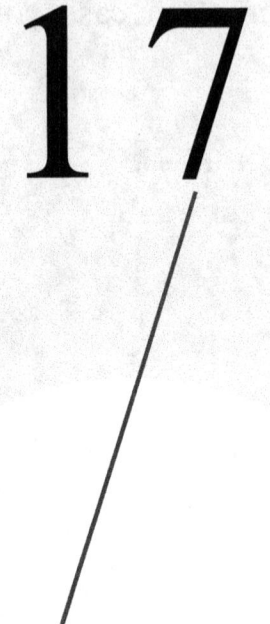

CHAPTER

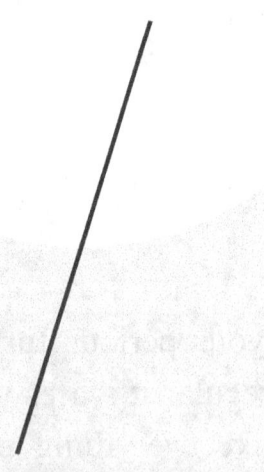

seventeen

Chapter Seventeen
Where are my tweezers?!

I don't know about you, but I seem to be losing the hair from my eyebrows, only to find them on my chin. I was a teenager in the 90s. My eyebrows are sparse, due to that amazing trend. I can't afford to lose anymore! Here is one thing that I know... those chin hairs can go pluck themselves.

There are two types of facial hair: Vellus hair is the short, soft, barely-there hair that children and women have. Terminal hair is longer, darker, thicker, and is generally found on men's faces.

Estrogen keeps hair finer, softer, and lighter. Darker, coarser, and thicker hair is a result of lower estrogen and higher testosterone. In Peri, estrogen diminishes, but women's testosterone may not. The higher ratio of testosterone to estrogen can cause those annoying chin hairs to sprout.

The good news is that if you can't find your tweezers, wax works. Laser treatment definitely works. Creams also work. Those annoying hairs are easy to get rid of. Personally, I love the wax strips. I heat them slightly with my hairdryer...

30 seconds later, the chin hair is gone.

Another symptom of Peri (and Meno) is hair loss. Although I've been lucky enough to not experience that kind of hair loss, except for my eyebrows, studies show that it is very common.

The British Association of Dermatologists looked at Peri/Meno women, 45 years and older of northern European descent. The results showed 41% of women had hair loss of some form.

26% experienced more generalized, all-over hair loss, while 9% had top of the scalp thinning.

In the study, 39% experienced increased facial hair with 32% of the group saying the hair was on the chin. *Ladies, I feel you.*

https://academic.oup.com/bjd/article-abstract/164/3/508/6644017

There's good news! Most menopausal women in the study also experienced loss of hair in the armpits, pubic area, and legs as they aged.

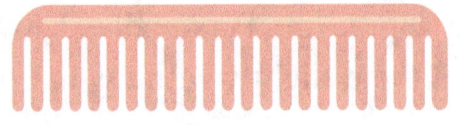

Side note - Tweezer tip... Leave a pair of tweezers in your car. The natural light, especially in broad daylight, is a perfect lighting for seeing where you need to pluck.
I shouldn't have to say this, but only do it when you're parked!

Hair loss during Peri/Meno is real! While it's normal to lose about 150 strands per day, losing more than that can be a sign of a deeper issue. If you find yourself losing a ton of hair, just to be on the safe side, see your physician. They can rule out things such as thyroid problems, anemia, or vitamin deficiencies.

Testosterone and other androgen hormones actually shrink the hair follicles on the scalp, making individual strands thinner. This can create an overall effect of thinning hair. Can you treat your hair loss at home? Absolutely! Using a volumizing shampoo and conditioner can add some thickness to your hair. Vitamin supplements can also be helpful, specifically Biotin. Biotin is an essential vitamin that promotes keratin formation for strong hair and nails.

Ladies... you aren't limited to at-home remedies.

There are very effective OTC medications that halt Meno hair loss like, Minoxidil (Rogaine). Rogaine is not just for men. Like most cosmetic treatments, they are also in-office hair loss solutions, such as PRP (platelet-rich plasma therapy).

One of the most frustrating things about Peri is that it isn't that your estrogen is gone, it's fluctuating. Sometimes your hair may look thick and healthy, and other times it may be thinner and lackluster.

Peri is a yo-yo. There seem to be a hundred different symptoms. Just when you think you've got a handle on it, it changes. Hair loss or chin hair gain are easily addressed at a salon or at home. Most, if not all of these symptoms are very normal. Hang in there. Chat with your doctor. Talk with your friends. Let's normalize these changes and stop hiding behind the fear, or shame of saying the words... perimenopause, period, vagina, estrogen, hair loss, mid-section weight gain, low sex drive, rage, or chin hair.

P.S. I hope you can find your tweezers!

18

CHAPTER

eighteen

Chapter Eighteen
Leaky gut, is that even a real thing?

First off, leaky gut? You would think that whoever came up with this term, could do better! I guess, I just don't like the word *guts.*

According to several sources, like my.clevelandclinic.org, Leaky gut syndrome is a theory and not necessarily a diagnosis, just yet.

Everyone's guts are semipermeable. The lining of our intestines is designed to absorb water and nutrients from things we ingest. Some people have increased intestinal permeability. That means that their guts are letting in more than water and nutrients.

Intestinal permeability is a recognized feature of several inflammatory and autoimmune diseases affecting the digestive system, including IBS and Celiac disease.

I think we all know that gut health is important, but what does it have to do with Peri?

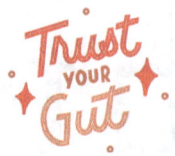

A leaky gut increases inflammation and compromises your body's ability to absorb nutrients. This can lead to hormonal imbalances, exacerbating the hormonal changes you're already experiencing due to Peri. The increased imbalance leads to increased Peri symptoms.

https://my.clevelandclinic.org/health/diseases/22724-leaky-gut-syndrome

It seems like gut health is something that we are learning more and more about, especially in recent years. Changing hormone levels, specifically falling estrogen, can significantly increase the risk of intestinal permeability. Estrogen normally helps to maintain a healthy intestinal barrier. It also thickens the mucus layer of the intestine.

Many scientists and doctors say that if you're suffering in the later phase of Peri with weight gain, digestive issues, mood symptoms, and fibromyalgia, consider whether intestinal permeability or leaky gut could be playing a role.

There's a growing body of evidence to suggest that the gut-hormone axis influences the amount of active estrogen circulating in your body.

During Peri, it looks like our gut microbiome gets disrupted by fluctuating estrogen levels. *What doesn't get disrupted?* The disruption of the microbiome may be directly associated with the common Peri symptoms we are all familiar with. These include increased IBS, bloating, hot flashes, weight gain, anxiety, brain fog, low energy, mood swings, loss of libido, vaginal dryness, urinary tract infections, and poor sleep. There are a lot of people that stand by this, somewhat new knowledge.

Many doctors have stated that in practice, by focusing on and improving gut health and supporting a diverse microbiome, many of the unwanted symptoms of Peri can be lessened.

Alexa — order probiotics

I'm sure there is merit to this evidence. It's logical. All I know is that I'm more constipated than I've ever been.

Like most symptoms of Peri, they come in waves. Right now, I'm on the constipated-insomnia wave. Are they related to each other, and does it have anything to do with gut health? It just might.

What can be done at home?
Mymenopausecentre.com breaks it down by saying,
"A healthy gut is very important (with or without Peri/Meno). Creating and maintaining good gut health is a daily task. It's not only our gut response to what we eat but also the response to our environment and our emotions. There's no cure that will solve all gut issues at once. There are some important daily habits that will make a huge impact.

Eat enough fiber. Fiber is essential for keeping our gut healthy. We need around 25g+ of fiber/day, but the average person only eats 15g. Ground flax seeds, onions, garlic, grains, beans, artichokes, leeks, bananas, and raspberries are all excellent sources of fiber."

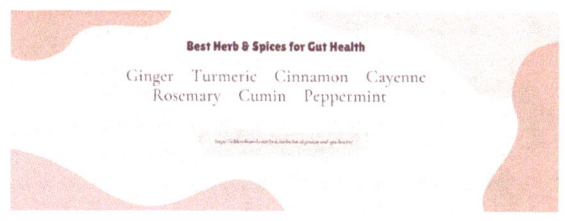

Best Herb & Spices for Gut Health

Ginger   Turmeric   Cinnamon   Cayenne
Rosemary   Cumin   Peppermint

"Probiotics will support the gut and liver, improving hormone balance, mood, sleep, digestion, and absorption.

Eat protein in every meal. We need protein to build hormones and neurotransmitters. 90% of the mood-boosting hormone, Serotonin, is made in our gut. We need to consume foods containing the amino acid tryptophan to support this process.

Eat good fats. We need good fats in our everyday diet to support better energy levels, hormone production, mood, skin, joint inflammation, and brain function. Good fat sources contain omega oils, which nourish our body inside and out. Foods, high in healthy fats are salmon, tuna, avocados, almonds, walnuts, pistachios, and pumpkin.

Move every day. Moving your body every day supports better gut mobility because when we exercise, the movements stimulate the muscles of our bowel wall. This can reduce constipation. Exercising or walking in the morning will get everything moving, boosting metabolism and energy throughout the day. Just 20 minutes makes a huge difference." *I need to do this!!*

"Lastly, manage stress. The gut-brain connection is an important link and when we experience stress, it causes our digestive system to slow down, as our body goes into fight or flight mode. This can have a negative impact on digestion and cause IBS-like symptoms. Whether it's yoga, meditation, or just taking a few minutes to breathe deeply throughout the day, this will all contribute to improving our stress resilience."

https://www.mymenopausecentre.com/blog/how-good-gut-health-can-improve-your-menopause-symptoms/

I think every one of us can agree that a person with a happy gut is also a happy person.

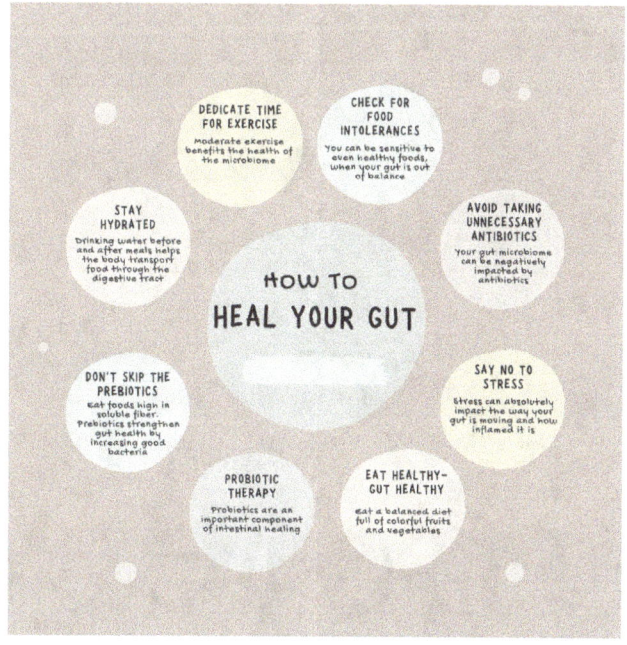

19

CHAPTER

nineteen

Chapter 19
Do I stay or do I go?

Do I stay or do I go?

Will it, or won't it?

Will my period come back? Or is it gone forever?

I think I asked myself those questions several times throughout my Peri adventure.
She really is a manipulative bitch. Just when you think that your time for bleeding is over, she shows back up again. Sometimes it's weeks, sometimes it's months.

In the beginning, I would curse her name because my periods were so close together. I would go two to three weeks between periods. That was four or five years ago.
Eventually, my cycle started spacing out. Pun intended. I would absolutely characterize Peri as spaced out.

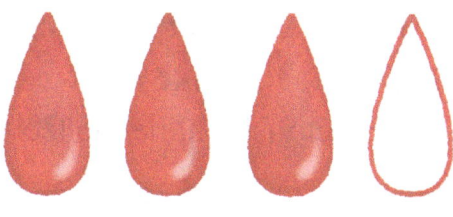

So, what should you expect? What I've learned through this whole process is that every woman is different. I've chatted with so many, and it seems like no two are the same. We all have our own Peri journey. Some are long, detailed, and gruesome. Some are short and easy, and I'm completely jealous of them!

Back to periods. Sometimes, in the middle of Peri, shit gets weird. Very, very weird. Month-to-month varies so drastically. You can go from having what seems like the longest and heaviest period of your life, followed by spotting for a few days.

This can go on for years. Years! What will the next month bring? I'm not going to lie to you. Those spotty months, or even those skipped months were a welcome change from those months that truly seemed like a murder scene.

Peri tip - have pregnancy tests on hand.

I knew I wasn't pregnant. Due to the irregularity, and sometimes absence of my period, I would check just to make sure. I think the negative test subconsciously made me feel more at ease.

Side note - Just stock up on the dollar store tests. It's a cheap and easy way to find peace of mind.

To sum things up, you never know what version of your period you're going to get each month. You could have the tiniest period, where you barely need any coverage. That's an awesome month.

Flip the coin... You might need to triple up on extra-large tampons, pads, and period underwear. You'll probably spend a ridiculous amount of time in the bathroom. How do men do it?

Always, always have a change of clothes.

Trust me on that one. Stash an extra pair of neutral pants in your car. You'll thank me. Oh! Also, stash an extra Ziploc bag, or a used grocery bag with these pants. You'll need to find a place to stow the bloody clothes.

Hindsight being 20/20, I did not do this. After a period blowout, I had an extra towel in my car. Thank goodness! I sat on it and quickly drove home. I was mortified.

My life became a waiting game. Every month made me wonder. Every month was different.

Two years before I finally stopped, my cycle was the most hostile. A violent period would show up and then months would go by. I would spot between periods and then realize - that was my period.

Finally, in February 2023, after a three-month sabbatical, I had a light period that lasted a few days.

March 2023 – Nothing

April 2023 – Nothing

May 2023 – Nothing

Is that it?
Of course not. Peri has to mess with me again.

My family had planned our first really big trip to France, Spain, Italy, and Greece. We flew into Paris and spent a quick, and glorious 36 hours there. We then hopped on a plane to Barcelona. Barcelona was our first port on the Mediterranean cruise.

I will never forget it. In the Charles Du Gaulle airport, I went to the Ladies room...

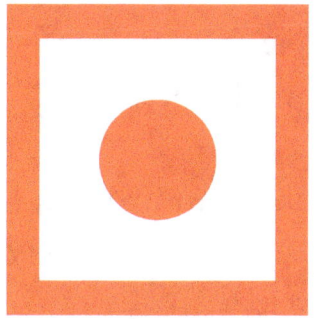

"You have got to be kidding me?!"
I wiped, and there was blood.
PUTAIN DE MERDE! This translates to something along the lines of, "fucking hell."
I remember thinking to myself, how do you say tampon in French? By the way, it is extremely difficult to find feminine products in a French airport.
After running around on a tampon search (at that point, I would've settled for a pad), I found some random, OB-like French tampons.

Oh, and the French word for tampon is:

le tampon

You never know when you will need that little tidbit of information.

We made it to Barcelona with no other problems. The next 24 hours were met with absolutely no blood. Not a drop.

And I haven't bled a day since. It was as if my period was saying, *Au revoir.*

It's fitting and unintentional, but today, as I write this chapter, it marks 365 days without any remnants of a cycle.

No spotting.

Nothing.

My gynecologist would later tell me that the "Paris period," was likely stress, combined with the tiniest bit of old uterine lining.

I thought the ending was poetic.

Welcome to Menopause.

P.S. I'm 47.

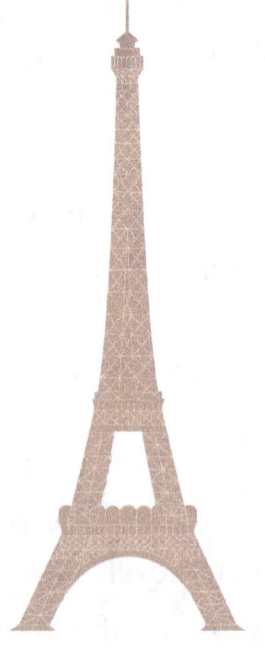

Your period and your body seem to be on the fritz. Why is this happening?

Peri may cause longer periods, shorter periods, and wacky periods. This is due to fluctuations in the hormones, specifically estrogen and progesterone.

According to verywellhealth.com, "During perimenopause, the hormones estrogen and progesterone can fluctuate wildly from month to month. If estrogen levels are higher than progesterone levels, the uterine lining can become thicker, and your body may take longer to shed it, leading to a longer period."

Because of hormone fluctuations, each month can be dramatically different from the month before.

These crazy hormone levels are also the culprit for spotting between periods.

https://www.verywellhealth.com/perimenopause-periods-5190945

You may have shorter cycles. During Peri, hormone levels change, which leads to a shorter follicular phase. When that happens, ovulation happens sooner.

The good news is that you're getting closer and closer to actual Meno. The bad news is that shorter cycles might mean you have two periods in one month. It's not as uncommon as you think.

You will probably experience heavier periods. When your estrogen levels are higher than your progesterone levels, the uterine lining grows, and that leads to more bleeding.

Side note - Don't be surprised when you skip periods, your following period is heavier, with more clots.

Do you know what people really don't talk about? No one talks about the emotional side of Peri. I'm not talking about moodiness, although there is a fair share of that! I'm talking about the feeling of loss. Maybe it's grieving because you can no longer bear children?

For me, it was bittersweet. I was ready. I was done with the fertile part of my life. Although part of me was, indeed, relieved, the other part of me was a little sad.

I think we grieve for what can never be? For what could have been?

I would've loved to have had a second child. It wasn't written in the stars for me and my husband and that's OK. I still wonder what it would be like. Sometimes, I feel the tiniest bit of guilt for not giving my daughter a sibling.

When I think about the idea of Menopause, I do feel the guilt. But I will also miss certain things.

I miss the estrogen!
It's kind of like a fountain of youth.
I miss collagen.
I miss my old sex drive.
I miss sleeping soundly.
I miss my old, perky boobs.
But I don't miss bleeding.
I certainly don't miss the anxiety
that comes along with the -
do I stay or do I go, part of Peri.

It was two years ago that my symptoms went from mild to moderate. Something else happened at that time. As I was leaving, or getting ready to leave the blood behind, my daughter was just starting.

It's either beautifully poetic or cosmically ironic.

Two years ago, we were like two emotional ships passing in the night. We were both experiencing the extreme highs and lows of erratic hormones.

My poor husband. He didn't know which way was up or down. It was around that time that he started kayak fishing more regularly.
Dear hubby... I get it!

I don't know about you, and whether you think it's poetic or ironic? I think it's a little bit of both.

I call it sweet serendipity.

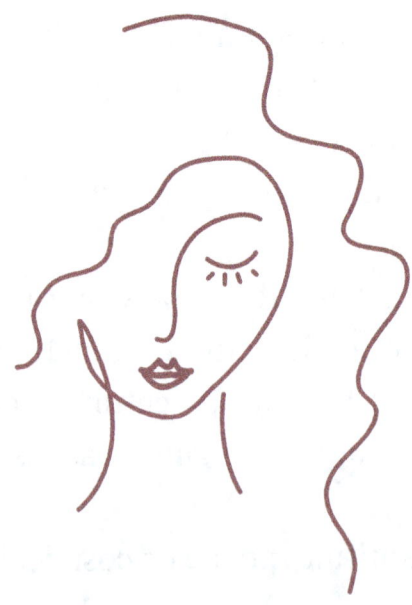

20

CHAPTER

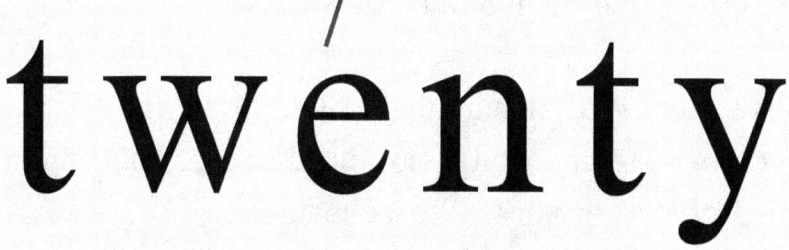
twenty

Chapter Twenty
Emotional Baggage?

Peri isn't just a bitch. I give her a hard time, but she's also an incredible teacher.

Throughout this journey, I have learned about myself, my wants, and my needs. Here are some other things that I've taken away from the entire experience.

Side note - Keep in mind, it's ongoing. You may even get a Volume 2: Meno Edition.

I've learned that I'm not alone. Most of the time, I have to be the starter of the conversation. I've found that if I bring up Peri or Meno, other ladies chime in. It's like they want to talk about it, but don't know how.

I've learned to always wear deodorant. Even if you think you don't need it, give yourself an underarm swipe. You never know when hot flashes are going to come. They can make you stinky.

I've learned that heightened emotions are OK. If you need to cry, cry! If you need to scream, scream in a pillow. It works like a charm!

I've learned that although my husband tries to understand, he just doesn't get it. I've also learned that he is a gem and loves me, even in those moments when I don't love myself. He's also oblivious to the age spots, weight gain, and all of those physical attributes that I see so clearly. He doesn't see them because they really aren't that obvious. I am just looking at myself from under a microscope.

I've learned to always keep tissues and underwear in my purse or in my car at all times. Trust me on this one. They will come in handy one day.

I've learned that most of us have unwanted chin hair. And I've learned that wax strips are super easy to use.

I've learned that it's OK to laugh at myself. In fact, I encourage it. Between the brain fog and the other wacky things going on with my body, sometimes they deserve a good laugh.

I've learned that throughout Meno, women should be tested for osteoporosis. Ask your doctor if you need or should have a bone scan.

I've learned that I can be an excellent source of knowledge and inspiration for friends and other women going through a similar journey.

I've learned that you can sleep wrong and throw out your back.

I'm in the process of learning that I'm still beautiful, and I'm still the person I used to be.

I've learned to give other ladies grace. When you see the woman fanning her face with a random object, she's in the thick of it.

I've learned that the only person that knows I'm peeing myself is me.

I've learned that things like retinol, hyaluronic acid, collagen, and other skin essentials are working overtime for me. Get your hands on some Tretinoin. It's worth every penny.

I've learned that my skin is more sensitive now. My skin used to soak up the sun. It still does, but I might get prickly heat, or I might get a few more sunspots.

I've learned that Find My Phone is an absolute godsend. I wish I could put an airtag on my glasses.

I've learned that I love not having a period.

I've learned that tacos and wine, separate or together, can turn a bad day into a good one.

I've learned to not judge people for their cosmetic procedures. Not sure I will ever do anything like that, but I get it. We all just want to feel pretty.

I've learned that even though I've turned into the family joke, chatting with my family about the side effects of Peri and Meno has brought us closer together. They are my best supporters.

I've learned that testing hormone levels can be pointless unless you have multiple tests, over a short period. Those tests measure your hormone levels at that moment. They will probably change the next day.

I've learned that insomnia comes and goes, but not sleeping will take its toll, emotionally.

I've learned that I am going to embrace my wrinkles. After all, they are from smiling, from frowning, and from some truly amazing memories.

I've learned that I am NOT going to embrace my rapidly graying hair. I'm still going to color the shit out of it.

I've learned that I'm not going to let my chest wrinkles, or what I call *chest stretch marks*, keep me from wearing a V-neck or a tank top. I've also learned that Go Pure Tighten & Lift Neck Cream works extremely well, for me.

I've learned that I definitely need readers, and that's OK.

I've also learned that I'm not going to shy away from the things that could hurt me, like playing tennis and enjoying the sun.

I've learned that it's easy to blame the big emotions on hormones. Sometimes, they are the root cause. Sometimes, Peri just gives you the assist to say what you've been dying to say.

I've learned that when traveling, be careful about my movie choice for in-flight entertainment. I will inevitably cry if it's too happy or too sad. "Top Gun, Maverick" is always a safe choice.

I've learned to master the art of the "Peri-Curtsy." Follow these steps... As you sneeze, hold yourself, and your bladder (from the inside). During the hold, cross your legs, as if doing a curtsy. It usually keeps the urine in.

I've learned that my joints ache. A lot. Diet helps.

I've learned that writing this book has been therapeutic. I've also learned that I've been spelling therapeutic wrong my entire life.

I've learned that Peri/Meno has some strange symptoms, symptoms I didn't mention.

I've learned that happiness is a choice, and I choose to be happy. You should too.

Thanks for reading.

QUESTIONS TO ASK
YOUR OB-GYN

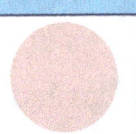

Instructions Come prepared for your next wellness visit. Make the best use of your appointment by having questions ready. Here are some examples.

Am I in Perimenopause? How do I know when I am in Menopause?

1

Should I use birth control during Perimenopause?

2

What are some signs or symptoms that I should expect as I enter Perimenopause?

3

Is my heavy bleeding normal?

4

What can I do about my insomnia and low libido?

5

What sort of supplements should I be taking?

6

Can I do anything about these hot flashes?

7

Are there lifestyle changes I should think about to ease my transition into Menopause?

8

What can you tell me about HRT? Am I a good candidate?

9

Do I need a pap smear every year?

10

What are the side effects of hormone therapy, and how does my individual health/family history affect my decision to take hormone therapy? What are the risks?

11

Can I do anything about these mood swings?

12

Based on my personal history, are there any other health concerns I need to know about, monitor and/or get screened for?

13

What should I know about bone health. Is a bone scan a routine test after Menopause?

14

What can I do to support my overall health and well-being?

15

Medical Disclaimer

This book details the author's personal experiences with and opinions about Perimenopause and Menopause. The author is not a [or your] healthcare provider. The author and publisher are providing this book and its contents on an "as is" basis and make no representations or warranties of any kind with respect to this book or its contents. The author and publisher disclaim all such representations and warranties, including for example warranties of merchantability and healthcare for a particular purpose. In addition, the author and publisher do not represent or warrant that the information accessible via this book is accurate, complete or current.

The contents of this book are not intended to diagnose, treat, cure, or prevent any condition or disease. Please consult with your own physician or healthcare specialist regarding the suggestions and recommendations made in this book. Except as specifically stated in this book, neither the author or publisher, nor any authors, contributors, or other representatives will be liable for damages arising out of or in connection with the use of this book. This is a comprehensive limitation of liability that applies to all damages of any kind, including (without limitation) compensatory; direct, indirect or consequential damages; loss of data, income or profit; loss of or damage to property and claims of third parties. You understand that this book is not intended as a substitute for consultation with a licensed healthcare practitioner, such as your physician. Before you begin any healthcare program, or change your lifestyle in any way, you will consult your physician or another licensed healthcare practitioner to ensure that you are in good health and that the examples contained in this book will not harm you.

This book provides content related to women's and/or sexual health issues. As such, use of this book implies your acceptance of this disclaimer.

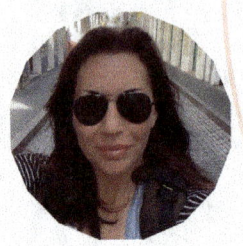

BIO

Angie Schwendeman is a wife, mother, photographer, and freelance writer. Born in 1977, this Cincinnati native resides in middle Georgia with her husband, daughter, and faithful black labrador. Although this is her first published book, she has been writing blogs, poetry, and stories since her days at The University of Tennessee, Knoxville. Go Big Orange!

She is a self-proclaimed wine snob who enjoys coffee, tennis, hummingbirds, travel, and spending time with her friends and family.

Stop by to say hello on Facebook or Instagram.

FB: www.facebook.com/profile.php?id=61565475286126
IG: www.instagram.com/angieschwendeman_author/

www.ingramcontent.com/pod-product-compliance
Lightning Source LLC
Chambersburg PA
CBHW071155130626
46553CB00004B/1674